Manual of Nephrology

Manual of
Nephrology

Richard S. Muther, M.D.

Medical Director, Nephrology
Research Medical Center
Kansas City, Missouri

John M. Barry, M.D.

Professor and Chairman
Division of Urology
Oregon Health Sciences University
Portland, Oregon

William M. Bennett, M.D.

Professor and Chairman
Division of Nephrology
Oregon Health Sciences University
Portland, Oregon

B.C. Decker Inc   Toronto ● Philadelphia

Publisher

B.C. Decker Inc
3228 South Service Road
Burlington, Ontario L7N 3H8

B.C. Decker Inc
320 Walnut Street
Suite 400
Philadelphia, Pennsylvania 19106

Sales and Distribution

United States and Puerto Rico
The C.V. Mosby Company
11830 Westline Industrial Drive
Saint Louis, Missouri 63146

Canada
McAinsh & Co. Ltd.
2760 Old Leslie Street
Willowdale, Ontario M2K 2X5

Australia
**McGraw-Hill Book Company Australia
Pty. Ltd.**
4 Barcoo Street
Roseville East 2069
New South Wales, Australia

Brazil
Editora McGraw-Hill do Brasil, Ltda.
rua Tabapua, 1.105, Itaim-Bibi
Sao Paulo, S.P. Brasil

Colombia
**Interamericana/McGraw-Hill de Colombia,
S.A.**
Apartado Aereo 81078
Bogota, D.E. Colombia

Europe
McGraw-Hill Book Company GmbH
Lademannbogen 136
D-2000 Hamburg 63
West Germany

France
MEDSI/McGraw-Hill
6, avenue Daniel Lesueur
75007 Paris, France

Hong Kong and China
McGraw-Hill Book Company
Suite 618, Ocean Centre
5 Canton Road
Tsimshatsui, Kowloon
Hong Kong

India
Tata McGraw-Hill Publishing Company, Ltd.
12/4 Asaf Ali Road, 3rd Floor
New Delhi 110002, India

Indonesia
P.O. Box 122/JAT
Jakarta, 1300 Indonesia

Italy
McGraw-Hill Libri Italia, s.r.l.
Piazza Emilia, 5
I-20129 Milano MI
Italy

Japan
Igaku-Shoin Ltd.
Tokyo International P.O. Box 5063
1-28-36 Hongo, Bunkyo-ku,
Tokyo 113, Japan

Korea
C.P.O. Box 10583
Seoul, Korea

Malaysia
No. 8 Jalan SS 7/6B
Kelana Jaya
47301 Petaling Jaya
Selangor, Malaysia

Mexico
**Interamericana/McGraw-Hill de Mexico,
S.A. de C.V.**
Cedro 512, Colonia Atlampa
(Apartado Postal 26370)
06450 Mexico, D.F., Mexico

New Zealand
McGraw-Hill Book Co. New Zealand Ltd.
5 Joval Place, Wiri
Manukau City, New Zealand

Panama
Editorial McGraw-Hill Latinoamericana, S.A.
Apartado Postal 2036
Zona Libre de Colon
Colon, Republica de Panama

Portugal
Editora McGraw-Hill de Portugal, Ltda.
Rua Rosa Damasceno 11A–B
1900 Lisboa, Portugal

South Africa
Libriger Book Distributors
Warehouse Number 8
"Die Ou Looiery"
Tannery Road
Hamilton, Bloemfontein 9300

Southeast Asia
McGraw-Hill Book Co.
348 Jalan Boon Lay
Jurong, Singapore 2261

Spain
**McGraw-Hill/Interamericana de Espana,
S.A.**
Manuel Ferrero, 13
28020 Madrid, Spain

Taiwan
P.O. Box 87–601
Taipei, Taiwan

Thailand
632/5 Phaholyothin Road
Sapan Kwai
Bangkok 10400
Thailand

United Kingdom, Middle East and Africa
McGraw-Hill Book Company (U.K.) Ltd.
Shoppenhangers Road
Maidenhead, Berkshire
SL6 2QL England

Venezuela
McGraw-Hill/Interamericana, C.A.
2da. calle Bello Monte
(entre avenida Casanova y Sabana Grande)
Apartado Aereo 50785
Caracas 1050, Venezuela

NOTICE

The authors and publisher have made every effort to ensure that the patient care recommended herein, including choice of drugs and drug dosages, is in accord with the accepted standards and practice at the time of publication. However, since research and regulation constantly change clinical standards, the reader is urged to check the product information sheet included in the package of each drug, which includes recommended doses, warnings, and contraindications. This is particularly important with new or infrequently used drugs.

Manual of Nephrology

ISBN 1-55664-048-X

Library of Congress catalog card number: 89-51033

10 9 8 7 6 5 4 3 2 1

Preface

This book was written by two nephrologists and a urologist for non-nephrologists. We thus apologize in advance for being too elementary for some while too esoteric for others.

Our major intent is to present a basic *diagnostic* approach to commonly encountered nephrologic problems. A recent survey of two large community hospitals identified such problems as those necessitating nephrology consultation (see Table). We discuss some of these problems generically (e.g., azotemia, proteinuria, and hematuria). Specific disease categories such as glomerulonephritis and interstitial nephritis are approached separately, even though proteinuria or hematuria may be their primary clinical manifestation.

Our discussion of these nephrologic problems is based on the assumption that most diagnostic failures occur because the clinician does not consider certain diseases or disease categories. In other words, diagnostic failures are the result of "omission, not commission." In order to minimize these failures, we present simplified methods for classifying various problems and diseases. Also presented are several simple diagnostic algorithms we have found useful.

Our method is based on four principles:

1. Once considered, a diagnosis is not difficult to confirm.
2. General categories of disease (e.g., glomerulonephritis or interstitial nephritis) should be considered before specific syndromes.

**The Distribution of Clinical Problems
Necessitating Nephrologic Consultation
in 298 Consecutive Cases**

	No. of Cases	% of Total Consultations
Azotemia	207	69
Acute	129	43
Postrenal	14	5
Prerenal	25	8
Renal paren-chymal	90	30
Chronic	78	26
Interstitial nephritis	34	11
Glomerulo-nephritis	24	8
Vascular disease	20	7
Hypertension	27	9
Proteinuria	20	7
Electrolyte distur-bance	8	3
Urinary tract infection	6	2
Hematuria	5	2
Nephrolithiasis	5	2
Acid-base abnormality	4	1
Other	16	5

3. Five (or fewer) diagnoses account for 95% of most disease categories ("Rule of Fives").
4. Diagnostic failures are minimized by considering the least likely diagnosis first.

In Chapter 1, we review the basic diagnostic tests (clinical, laboratory, and radiographic) that are most useful in assessing renal structure and function. Chapters 2 through 12 discuss the major clinical problems in nephrology.

At the beginning of each chapter, we present cases as unknowns. We encourage the reader to answer the "prechapter" questions and generate a differential diagnosis based on the information provided for each case. A brief review of each topic follows. Although this review touches upon the pertinent epidemiology, pathophysiology, and therapy for each condition, the major emphasis is on a diagnostic approach distilled from the basic information. Subsequently, each case is reviewed and the prechapter questions answered.

The text is not encyclopedic, nor do we consider the coverage of pathophysiology and therapeutics adequate for clinical practice. In addition, discussions of chronic renal failure and hypertension are omitted. To compensate for this, we refer the reader to several excellent review and reference texts.

Richard S. Muther, M.D.
John M. Barry, M.D.
William M. Bennett, M.D.

Contents

1 Clinical Evaluation of Renal Structure and
   Function | 1

2 Asymptomatic Urinary Abnormalities | 25

3 Acute Renal Failure | 53

4 Glomerulonephritis | 89

5 Interstitial Nephritis | 131

6 Vascular Disease of the Kidney | 157

7 Clinical Disorders of Sodium Balance: Derangements of
   the Extracellular Volume | 183

8 Clinical Disorders of Water Balance: Hyponatremia and
   Hypernatremia | 213

9 Clinical Disorders of Potassium Balance | 237

10 Metabolic Acid-Base Disorders | 259

11 Urinary Tract Infection Syndromes | 283

12 Nephrolithiasis | 297

   Index | 317

1 Clinical Evaluation of Renal Structure and Function

- Imaging Techniques for the Genitourinary Tract

- Clinical Evaluation of the Glomerulus

- Clinical Evaluation of the Tubules and Interstitium

This initial chapter is divided into three parts discussing (1) imaging tests, (2) tests used to evaluate the glomerulus, and (3) tests used to evaluate the tubules and interstitium. This is in keeping with our general principle of considering major disease categories (e.g., glomerulonephritis or interstitial nephritis) before considering specific clinical syndromes in the diagnosis of nephrologic problems.

Imaging Techniques for the Genitourinary Tract

Table 1-1 lists commonly used imaging techniques and their relative merits in evaluating renal structure and function. Although the plain *abdominal film* (KUB) provides little specific information, it is commonly available and has benefits that should be emphasized. Renal size and shape are usually evident on KUB, particularly if nephrotomography is used. Ascites and psoas obliteration suggesting abscess, hematoma, or tumor can also be seen on plain

Table 1-1 Relative Merit (0–4+) of Common Imaging Techniques in the Assessment of Renal Structure and Function

	Structure	*Function*	*Comment*
KUB	1+	0	Gross structural change evident. Good for following nephrolithiasis.
IVP with voiding and postvoid films	3+	3+	Best for simultaneous evaluation of structure and function of entire genitourinary tract. Limited by renal function impairment.
Retrograde pyelography	4+	1+	Best for anatomic delineation of ureters, pelvis, and calyces.
Cystography	3+	2+	Best for anatomic delineation of bladder. Voiding urethrogram enhances evaluation of lower urinary tract. May outline ureters if reflux is present.
Ultrasonography	3+	0	Noninvasive, low-risk. Best screening test for structural abnormalities.
CT	4+	2+	Has better resolution than ultrasonography. Can be used without contrast to exclude obstruction. Dynamic study with contrast can yield function information.
Radionuclide scanning ^{131}I-Hippuran ^{99m}Tc-DTPA	1+	3+	Sensitive but nonspecific. Evaluates tubular secretion and renal excretion. Evaluates renal blood flow.

Table 1-1 (Continued)

	Structure	*Function*	*Comment*
Indium			When tagged to white blood cells can local-ize renal infection.
Arteriography	4+	4+	Gold standard. Should be reserved for confirma-tion of specific lesion.

film. Free peritoneal, retroperitoneal, or intraurinary tract gas can likewise be detected, suggesting viscus perforation or gas-forming bacterial infection. Finally, abnormal calcification of bone (osteo-dystrophy, lytic or sclerotic lesions), renal parenchyma (nephro-calcinosis), or collecting system (nephrolithiasis, ureterolithiasis, or cystolithiasis) can be assessed by KUB. The latter is particularly useful in the serial evaluation of nephrolithiasis.

The abdominal plain film is greatly enhanced by administering intravenous (IV) contrast material excreted by the kidney. Such an excretory urogram (XU) or *intravenous pyelogram (IVP)* highlights the renal parenchyma, and better delineates renal size and shape. Renal cysts and tumors are thus more easily seen. Concentration of contrast material in the collecting system (5 to 15 minutes after injection) outlines the calyces, renal pelvis, ureters, and bladder (Fig. 1-1) allowing definition of genitourinary tumors, calculi, ob-struction, and chronic pyelonephritis. Films taken early (1 minute after injection) can be used to evaluate differential renal perfusion (hypertensive IVP) and are often used as a screening test for reno-vascular hypertension (see Chapter 2).

Unfortunately, the IVP is limited by potential contrast toxicity in three forms: minor allergic reactions (hives, pruritus), anaphylactic reactions, and nephrotoxicity (see Chapter 3). Renal insufficiency may fail to allow excretion and concentration of contrast material, further limiting the value of the IVP. This latter problem can be minimized by using nephrotomography (Fig. 1-2) and a greater

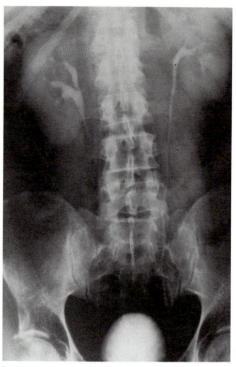

Figure 1-1: *A*, Normal IVP outlining the kidneys, ureters, and bladder.

A

dose of IV contrast, although this will increase the potential for nephrotoxicity.

Although the IVP is neither the most sensitive nor the most specific renal imaging study, it has the advantage of providing both structural and functional information on the entire urinary tract and is therefore an excellent screening test.

When renal insufficiency is severe enough to limit the IVP, a *retrograde pyelogram* or *cystogram* is used to evaluate the renal pelvis, ureters, or bladder. A retrograde pyelogram can definitively exclude obstruction and evaluate filling defects (Fig. 1-3). A cystogram allows specific definition of bladder outlet obstruction, vesicoureteral reflux, trauma, diverticula, or fistula (Fig. 1-4). When

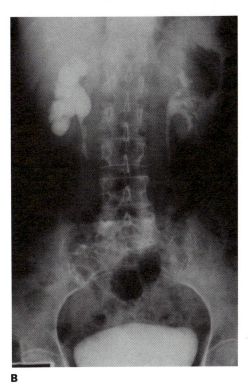

B

Figure 1-1: *B*, IVP showing right ureteral obstruction.

used with a voiding study (*cystourethrogram*), urethral strictures, urethral diverticula, posterior urethral valves, and bladder-emptying are also defined.

The renal *ultrasonogram* offers a noninvasive and relatively low-cost way of evaluating the kidney without the risk of IV contrast (Fig. 1-5). Renal size, cysts, tumors, hydronephrosis, and stones are all well defined by sonography. Its accuracy in determining renal size and excluding obstruction makes it the initial screening test for evaluation of azotemia.

Computed tomography (CT) offers better resolution than ultrasonography and enables one to make a definitive diagnosis of a renal mass, often eliminating the need for cyst puncture and/or arte-

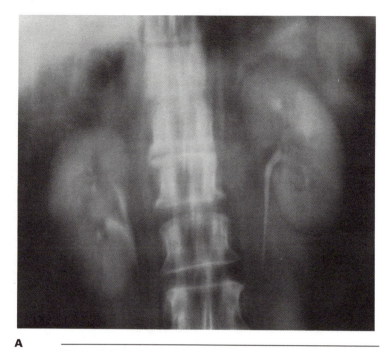

A

Figure 1-2: *A*, Accentuation of renal cortex and calyces by the use of nephrotomography with the IVP.

riography (Fig. 1-6). It can also be used without IV contrast to exclude obstruction in the azotemic patient and to define retroperitoneal, adrenal, and perirenal architecture. Yet despite these advantages, CT is more cumbersome and costly than ultrasonography and therefore usually assumes a secondary role in diagnosis.

Several radionucleotide scans offer information on renal function. *Hippuran* is secreted by renal tubular cells, and when it is tagged with radioactive ^{131}I, one can evaluate renal tubular function and excretion through the lower urinary tract. It is used primarily as a predictor of renal tubular recuperation after acute tubular necrosis or as a means of defining the relative contribution of each kidney to

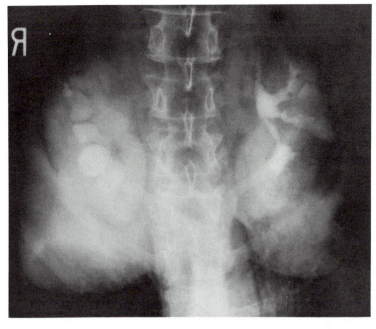

Figure 1-2: *B*, Nephrotomography in a patient with right ureteral obstruction.

total renal function. *Technetium-99m* (^{99m}Tc)-tagged diethylenetri-
amine penta-acetic acid (DTPA) offers a sensitive estimate of renal
blood flow. Unfortunately, both of these studies lack specificity, so
that an IVP, CT, or ultrasonogram is usually necessary for evaluating morphology, and arteriography is usually necessary for definitive assessment of the renal circulation in patients with focal or
unilateral perfusion defects by scan.

An indium-tagged white blood cell (WBC) study may often
localize an occult infection process in the kidney. It offers equal
sensitivity but greater specificity than gallium-67 which is not specific for infection.

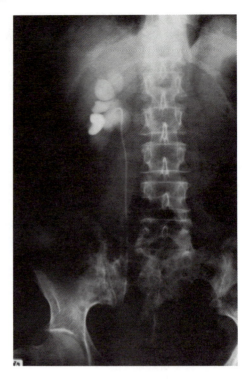

Figure 1-3: Right retrograde pyelogram in a patient with ureteropelvic junction obstruction.

Renal *arteriography* is the most sensitive and specific test to evaluate renal vascular structure (Figs. 1-7A and B). It is the definitive test for evaluating renal vascular lesions and the renal mass. It can also be used for specific therapeutic intervention such as balloon angioplasty for renal artery stenosis or renal ablation by embolization or thrombosis (Fig. 1-7C). Risks include those of arterial puncture, those incurred by IV contrast, and the possibility of traumatizing an atherosclerotic aorta or renal artery, causing distal atheroemboli.

Table 1-2 presents a problem-oriented approach to renal imaging techniques used as screening (most sensitive) and confirmatory (most specific) tests. For patients with hematuria, the IVP visualizes

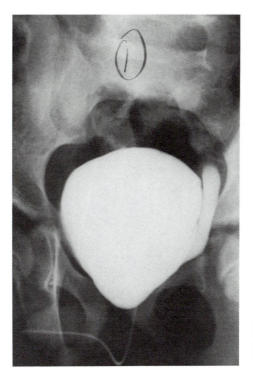

Figure 1-4: Cystogram demonstrating left ureteral reflux.

the entire urinary tract. If the cause of hematuria is not readily apparent, cystoscopy and perhaps retrograde pyelography are indicated. CT or arteriography will be needed to evaluate any renal mass. IVP is also the best screening test to use in patients with non-nephrotic–range proteinuria to evaluate potential parenchymal disease (e.g., vesicoureteral reflux, chronic pyelonephritis, renal tuberculosis, amyloid, and cystic diseases). If the IVP is negative, further radiographic studies are probably not warranted. When using IVP as a screening test in these patients, one must consider the potential for contrast toxicity and define those at high risk (patients with diabetes, myeloma, and/or renal insufficiency).

In the azotemic patient, renal ultrasonography offers clear ad-

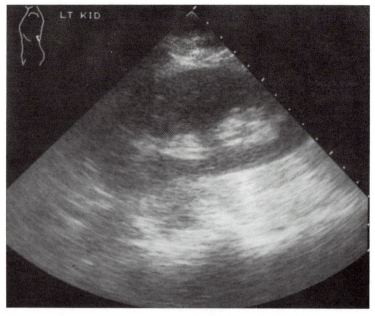

Figure 1-5: *A*, Normal renal ultrasonography. Note that renal cortex is more lucent than the background. Medulla and papillae are echogenic.

vantages as a screening test. Acutely, a ^{99m}Tc-DTPA nucleotide scan can exclude a gross abnormality of renal perfusion. If there is such an abnormality, an arteriogram may be required for definitive diagnosis. A retrograde pyelogram can similarly specify the cause of any obstruction noted by initial ultrasonography.

Because IVP can evaluate renal perfusion, asymmetric renal size, obstruction, and renal parenchymal disease, it is the procedure of choice when one is screening for renal causes of secondary hypertension. If one is specifically concerned about renovascular hypertension, equal support can be generated for ^{99m}Tc-DTPA nucleotide scanning and venous digital subtraction angiography (DSA) as screening tests. Often, however, screening for renovascular disease

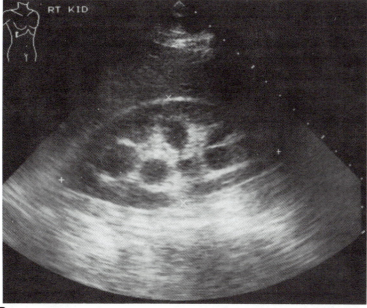

Figure 1-5: *B*, Renal ultrasonography demonstrating obstruction. Note displacement of central echoes by caliectasis. *Figure continues on following page.*

is performed during the history and physical examination, and a more specific test is warranted (see Chapter 2).

An IVP is indicated in patients with recurrent lower urinary tract infections, pyelonephritis, or genitourinary sepsis in order to exclude anatomic defects. A renal ultrasonogram can be used in azotemic patients. The same approach applies to patients with suspected urinary tract obstruction.

Ultrasonography and CT should be all that is necessary to differentiate a cystic mass from a solid renal mass, thus eliminating the need for cyst puncture. An arteriogram may be necessary if doubt remains regarding the diagnosis and/or if anatomic definition of the renal vasculature is required before surgery.

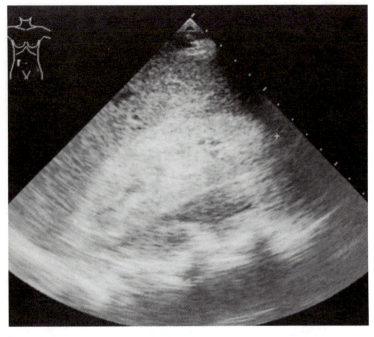

C

Figure 1-5 (Continued): *C*, Renal ultrasonography demonstrating markedly increased echogenicity of the renal parenchyma in a patient with AIDS nephropathy.

Clinical Evaluation of the Glomerulus

The major functions of the renal glomeruli are (1) filtering the blood of various wastes (e.g., urea and creatinine) and (2) retaining protein and blood cells as filtration occurs. Diseases that primarily affect the renal glomerulus are therefore manifest as an abnormality (usually a decrement) in the rate of glomerular filtration or an inappropriate loss of protein in the urine (Fig. 1-8).

The glomerular filtration rate (GFR) is measured by several methods. The most accurate of these is the clearance of inulin (C_{in}).

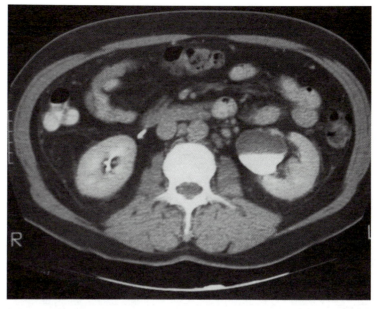

A

Figure 1-6: *A*, CT scan showing left renal obstruction. Note contrast "level" in left renal pelvis. *Figure continues on following page.*

Inulin (with a molecular weight of 5,000) is freely filtered by the renal glomerulus and undergoes neither tubular reabsorption nor secretion. Its rate of appearance in the urine is therefore completely determined by the filtration rate of the renal glomeruli and is expressed by the *clearance formula:*

$$C_{in} \ (ml/min) \ = \ \frac{U_{in} \ (mg/dl) \cdot vol \ (ml/min)}{P_{in} \ (mg/dl)}$$

where U_{in} equals urinary inulin, vol equals urinary volume, and P_{in} equals the steady-state plasma inulin concentration. Because inulin is an exogenous substance, an inulin infusion is necessary to perform this test. This limits its clinical applicability.

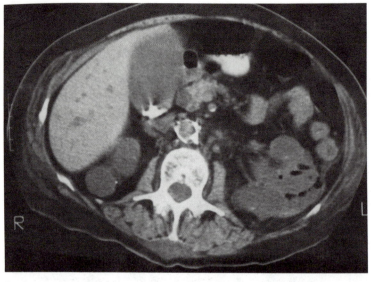

B

Figure 1-6 (Continued): *B*, CT scan in a patient with polycystic kidney disease. Note the presence of gas in the left kidney, indicating infection.

Clinically, glomerular filtration is best measured by the endogenous creatinine clearance (C_{cr}). Creatinine is produced by the conversion of muscle creatine in the liver and is excreted in the urine. Because the renal excretion (clearance) of creatinine is roughly equal to its production, the plasma creatinine (P_{cr}) remains relatively constant. Therefore, no IV infusion is necessary to perform the creatinine clearance, which is:

$$C_{cr} \text{ (ml/min)} = \frac{U_{cr} \text{ (mg/dl)} \cdot \text{vol (ml/min)}}{P_{cr}}$$

Over wide ranges of glomerular filtration, the C_{cr} closely approximates the C_{in} and can be substituted for GFR in clinical practice.

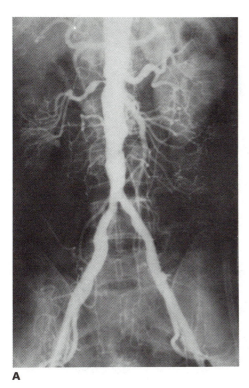

A

Figure 1-7: *A,* Aortogram showing right renal artery stenosis. *Figure continues on following page.*

Two peculiarities of the C_{cr} may affect its proper interpretation. The first of these is renal tubular creatinine secretion, which accounts for roughly 20% of excreted creatinine (80% being filtered). Thus, 20% of the creatinine that appears in the urine has not undergone filtration, a fact which, when overlooked, can cause GFR to be overestimated. Fortunately, this is offset by the second peculiarity—an imperfection in the usual plasma creatinine assay (Jaffé reaction) which "overmeasures" true plasma creatinine by roughly 20% (resulting in a higher plasma creatinine and an underestimation of GFR). Because these defects are qualitatively opposite and of equal magnitude, they in effect cancel each other out and allow for the close correlation of C_{cr} and C_{in}.

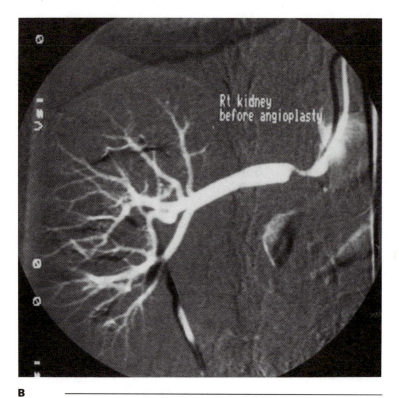

B

Figure 1-7 (Continued): *B*, Renal arteriogram demonstrating right renal artery stenosis.

Occasionally, however, a drug may compete for tubular creatinine secretion. Alternatively, certain drugs and chemicals are measured as creatinine in the plasma by the chemical assay. Each of these phenomena would spuriously elevate plasma creatinine and underestimate GFR. Substances responsible for this artifactual rise in creatinine and which should be kept in mind are trimethoprim and cimetidine (substances competing for tubular creatinine secre-

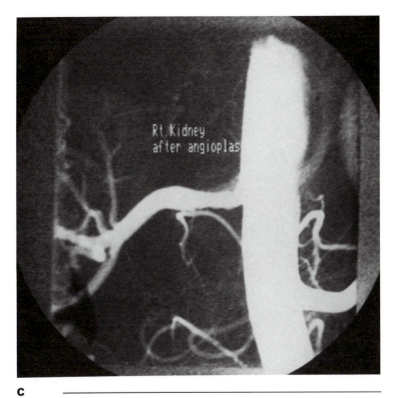

Figure 1-7: *C*, Renal arteriogram in same patient after balloon angioplasty.

tion) and cefoxitin and acetone (substances incorrectly measured as creatinine).

Another potential disadvantage of the C_{cr} is that it necessitates a timed (usually 24-hour) urine collection. Incomplete urine collections usually lead to errors in C_{cr}. These can be checked by confirming that the daily urinary creatinine excretion (mg/24 hr) approximates the daily creatinine production (15 to 20 mg/kg/day in

Table 1-2 Problem-Oriented Approach to Renal Imaging Techniques

Problem	Radiograph Screening	Radiograph Confirmation	Comment
Hematuria	IVP	Cystoscopy-retrograde pyelogram	For use if cause of hematuria is not apparent.
		CT	To evaluate renal mass.
Proteinuria	IVP	Variable	Primarily to evaluate non-nephrotic–range proteinuria.
Acute azotemia	Ultrasonography ^{99m}Tc-DTPA	Retrograde pyelogram Arteriogram	Primarily necessary to exclude obstruction and assess gross blood flow.
Chronic azotemia	Ultrasonography	CT	Small, non-obstructed kidneys rarely require confirmatory study.
Hypertension	IVP (^{99m}Tc-DTPA, DSA)*	Arteriogram	Clinical setting determines the work-up for renovascular disease*
	CT		CT excludes adrenal or retroperitoneal tumors.

Table 1-2 (Continued)

| Problem | Radiograph | | Comment |
	Screening	Confirmation	
Urinary tract infection	IVP	CT	To exclude intra- or peri- nephric abscess.
	Ultrasonography[†]	Cystogram	To exclude ves- icoureteral reflux or bladder out- let obstruc- tion.
		Indium	May detect oc- cult abscess.
Renal mass	Ultrasonography	CT	To differentiate cystic masses from solid masses.
		Arteriogram	To exclude malig- nancy, arte- riovenous malforma- tion.
Obstruction	IVP	CT	Allows assess- ment of retroperi- toneum.
	Ultrasonography†	Retrograde pyelogram	Allows definitive localization; often diag- nostic; possi- ble drainage.
		Antegrade pyelo- gram	Can be used when retro- grade impos- sible.

* See discussion of renovascular hypertension in Chapter 2.
† If patient is azotemic, ultrasonography is preferred to avoid IV contrast.

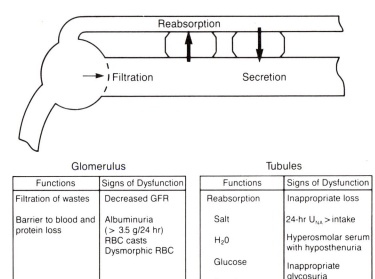

Glomerulus	
Functions	Signs of Dysfunction
Filtration of wastes	Decreased GFR
Barrier to blood and protein loss	Albuminuria (> 3.5 g/24 hr) RBC casts Dysmorphic RBC

Tubules	
Functions	Signs of Dysfunction
Reabsorption	Inappropriate loss
Salt	24-hr U_{NA} > intake
H_2O	Hyperosmolar serum with hyposthenuria
Glucose	Inappropriate glycosuria
Proteins	Globulinuria (> 200 mg/day)
Secretion	Failure to secrete
H^+	Hyper Cl acidosis
K^+	Hyperkalemia
Uric Acid	Hyperuricemia

Figure 1-8: The functions (and signs of dysfunction) of the glomerulus and tubules which offer clinical diagnostic clues to glomerulonephritis or tubulointerstitial nephritis.

women; 20 to 25 mg/kg/day in men). Failure to achieve these levels of urinary creatinine invalidates the C_{cr}, regardless of the degree of renal function impairment.

Using the plasma creatinine alone as a marker for GFR eliminates the need for quantitative urine collections. Figure 1-9 shows

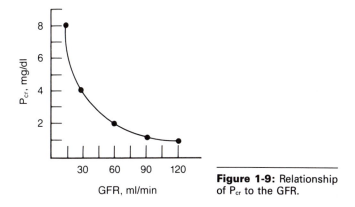

Figure 1-9: Relationship of P_{cr} to the GFR.

the inverse relationship between the plasma creatinine and the C_{cr} (a similar curve can be drawn for blood urea). Because of this reciprocal relationship, $1 \div P_{cr}$ is often plotted over time to follow the course of various renal diseases (Fig. 1-10). The GFR can also be estimated from P_{cr} by several formulae, the most simple of which is:

$$GFR = \frac{Body\ weight\ (kg)}{P_{cr}}$$

when the GFR is less than 50 ml/min.

It is important to remember that all methods relying on P_{cr} as a measure of GFR depend on a stable steady-state P_{cr}. If creatinine production is changing (e.g., with rhabdomyolysis) or creatinine excretion has acutely declined (e.g., with acute renal failure), the P_{cr} inaccurately reflects the GFR. One must also remember that P_{cr} is dependent on muscle mass. Thus a 24-hour C_{cr} is recommended initially to properly correlate the P_{cr} to the GFR.

Glomerular dysfunction is measured not only by a decrement in filtration but also by a loss of the filtration barrier. Normally, the filtration of proteins across the glomerular capillary membrane is limited by size and charge (see Chapter 2). In the absence of disease, proteins with molecular weights greater than 60,000 and

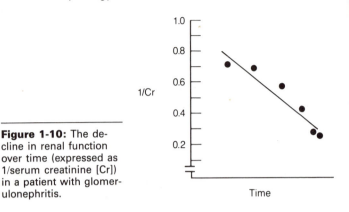

Figure 1-10: The decline in renal function over time (expressed as 1/serum creatinine [Cr]) in a patient with glomerulonephritis.

those which are negatively charged do not cross the filtration barrier. Albumin, for example (with a molecular weight of 60,000; negatively charged), is usually not filtered. Only positively charged globulins of low molecular weight usually cross and appear in the urine (<2 g daily filtered, <200 mg daily excreted). With glomerular disease however, this barrier is disrupted and albumin is easily detected in the urine. Thus albuminuria (by electrophoresis) or massive proteinuria (>3.5 g/day) are considered diagnostic of glomerular disease.

Another sign of glomerular capillary disruption is of course hematuria, especially if one can document in the urine sediment red blood cell (RBC) casts or the dysmorphic RBC ascribed to glomerular disease (see Chapter 2).

Clinical Evaluation of the Tubules and Interstitium

The two major functions of the renal tubules are (1) reabsorption of most of the glomerular filtrate and (2) secretion of various molecules, most notably hydrogen ion and potassium. Failure of appropriate reabsorption and/or secretion is therefore indicative of tubular dysfunction and can be detected by a variety of clinical tests.

The *urinary sodium* (U_{NA}) is an excellent indicator of tubular reabsorptive capacity when the patient's total sodium balance is considered. In a normal individual (not gaining or losing weight), sodium excretion equals sodium intake—i.e., the person eating 150 mEq of sodium daily should excrete 150 mEq in the urine daily. If the patient is significantly volume-contracted, however, renal tubular sodium reabsorption should increase and U_{NA} should decrease, usually to less than 10 mEq daily or approximately 20 mEq/L. In the volume-contracted patient, a high U_{NA} (<20 mEq/L) therefore indicates a failure in reabsorption and likely signifies tubular dysfunction or disease (e.g., acute tubular necrosis).

The sensitivity of the U_{NA} can be markedly enhanced by the fractional excretion of Na (FE_{NA}). The FE_{NA} is the fraction of the sodium filtered (plasma sodium $\times$ GFR), which is ultimately excreted and is calculated as follows:

$$FE_{NA} = \frac{\text{Sodium excreted}}{\text{Sodium filtered}}$$

$$= \frac{U_{NA} \text{ (meq/L)} \cdot \text{vol}}{P_{NA} \text{ (mEq/L)} \cdot \dfrac{U_{cr} \text{ (mg/dl)} \cdot \text{vol}}{P_{cr} \text{ (mg/dl)}}} \times 100$$

$$= \frac{U_{NA}/P_{NA}}{U_{cr}/P_{cr}} \times 100$$

where P_{NA} equals plasma sodium.

In reality, the FE_{NA} is the opposite of the fractional reabsorption of sodium and therefore an excellent indicator of tubular reabsorption; as the tubular reabsorption of sodium increases, the FE_{NA} falls, whereas a decrease in sodium reabsorption increases FE_{NA}. (The importance of the U_{NA} and FE_{NA} in the differential diagnosis of the acutely azotemic patient is elaborated in Chapter 3.)

Like sodium, failure to reabsorb filtered water is another sign of tubular dysfunction. Failure to reabsorb water is manifest as hyposthenuria (low urinary osmolarity [U_{osm}] or specific gravity) in the face of plasma hyperosmolarity. If the plasma osmolarity is greater than 290 mOsm/L but the U_{osm} is less than 300 mOsm/L, one can assume inappropriate water loss or diabetes insipidus (DI). In the presence of antidiuretic hormone (ADH) (central DI excluded), this water loss indicates significant tubular dysfunction (nephrogenic DI). The urine-specific gravity correlates with the osmolarity but can be influenced by glycosuria and proteinuria and is therefore less accurate than the U_{osm}.

Because plasma sodium is the major component of plasma osmolarity, hypernatremia is often a sign of pathologic water loss as well (see Chapter 8).

Occasionally, inappropriate loss of urinary protein (Fanconi's syndrome) and glucose is caused by tubular reabsorptive failure. In most patients, glucosuria is considered inappropriate if the simultaneous serum glucose is less than 160 mg/dl.

Tubular dysfunction is also suggested by failure to secrete hydrogen ion (H^+) and potassium (K^+) appropriately. In patients with renal insufficiency, plasma K^+ is usually maintained within the normal range until the GFR is extremely low (<5 ml/min). A similarly low GFR is required before uremic acidosis occurs, raising the anion gap. However, hyperkalemia and H^+ ion retention can occur despite relative preservation of GFR (C_{cr} = 15 to 30 ml/minute; P_{cr} = 1.5 to 5 mg/dl) if tubular ion secretion is impaired. In this setting, hyperkalemia and a hyperchloremic (non-anion gap) metabolic acidosis are often seen.

Thus the plasma electrolytes (Na, K, Cl, HCO_3) may be important indicators of renal tubular dysfunction and should be considered carefully.

The urinary sediment may also provide clues to tubular and/or interstitial inflammation. Generally, pyuria predominates over hematuria, although both may be observed. Even in the absence of infection, pyuria is still evident in most patients with interstitial nephritis (see Chapter 5). WBC and renal tubular cell casts can also be seen with sterile urine in a variety of interstitial nephropathies.

The above-described abnormalities may be very useful in the attempt to differentiate glomerular from interstitial disease (see Chapter 2).

2   Asymptomatic Urinary Abnormalities

- Case Presentations
- Hematuria
- Proteinuria
- Azotemia
- Hypertension
- Case Discussions

Case 2-1

A 26-year-old woman had gross hematuria during a febrile illness characterized by sore throat and cervical adenopathy. Urinalysis confirmed hematuria and identified 2 + proteinuria. Blood urea nitrogen (BUN) and serum creatinine levels were normal. Although the gross hematuria and proteinuria resolved, microscopic hematuria persisted. When seen 6 weeks later, she had 15 to 20 RBCs per high power field (RBC/hpf). Surface irregularities were noted on all of the RBCs. Blood pressure was 112/28. Physical examination normal.

Questions

1. What is the most likely cause of the hematuria?
2. What further tests are indicated?

Case 2-2

A 67-year-old man had four episodes of total, gross, painless hematuria over a 12-hour period. (Seven years earlier, he underwent a transurethral prostatectomy and transurethral removal of bladder stones.) Physical examination, including vital signs, was normal. Dipstick urinalysis showed a pH of 6, no protein, sugar, bilirubin, leukocyte esterase, or nitrites, and trace blood. Microscopic urinalysis showed three to five RBC/hpf. None of the RBCs were dysmorphic (i.e., with surface irregularities).

Questions

1. What diagnostic steps are appropriate to evaluate this patient's hematuria?

Case 2-3

A 30-year-old woman complaining of fatigue and weakness had 2+ urinary protein by dipstick on several occasions over a 4-week period. The urinalysis was otherwise normal. (Nine months earlier, she had a petechial rash diagnosed by a dermatologist as "cutaneous vasculitis." It resolved when treated with corticosteroids. An ANA was negative at that time.) Physical examination was normal, and blood pressure was 114/76. The hemoglobin was 13.1; WBC count was 3.3; platelets were normal. A 24-hour urine collection showed a creatinine clearance of 117 ml/min and urine protein of 898 mg.

Questions

1. What diagnostic steps are appropriate to evaluate this patient's proteinuria?

Case 2-4

During an evaluation for hypertension, a 54-year-old woman was found to have a BUN of 42 mg/dl and a serum creatinine of 3.2 mg/dl. She had not seen a physician since she was treated for ulcers 10 years earlier. She had no known history of renal disease, hematuria, proteinuria, nephrolithiasis, or urinary infection. Except for experiencing chronic headaches, she did not feel weak. Except for mild hypertension, her physical examination was normal.

Laboratory evaluation further revealed hemoglobin of 9.7 g/dl; serum sodium was 137 mEq/L; potassium, 5.7 mEq/L; chloride, 114 mEq/L; and bicarbonate, 14 mEq/L. The urinalysis revealed pH of 5.0, 1+ proteinuria, three to five RBC/hpf and eight to ten WBC/hpf. No casts were seen. A 24-hour urine collection showed a urine protein of 1,100 mg. The creatinine clearance was 20 ml/min.

Questions

1. Does the patient have acute or chronic azotemia?
2. What test(s) can be used to confirm your suspicion?
3. What type of renal parenchymal disease (glomerular, interstitial, or vascular) do you now suspect? What etiology?

Case 2-5

A 53-year-old woman presented with dyspnea. Initial blood pressure was 194/118 without orthostatic change. She related a history of high blood pressure of several years' standing treated with a variety of medications, but had not taken blood pressure pills for the last 3 years. Her medical history was otherwise negative. Both her mother and one sibling had hypertension. Physical examination showed trace edema, absence of an abdominal bruit, and minimal (Grade I) retinopathy, but was otherwise normal. Laboratory tests revealed a normal urinalysis, normal complete blood count (CBC) and normal serum chemistries (with the exception of a serum potassium of 2.8 mEq/L and bicarbonate of 30 mEq/L.

Questions

1. Is further evaluation needed before treatment?
2. What is the most likely cause of secondary hypertension in this patient?

Any renal disease may be asymptomatic, particularly if it is chronic and slowly evolving. In this chapter, we focus on those diseases often presenting as isolated abnormalities—namely, hematuria, proteinuria, azotemia, and hypertension. (Pyuria is explored in Chapter 11.)

Hematuria

Hematuria (>1 RBC/hpf in males; >3 RBC/hpf in females) is usually of urologic, not nephrologic, origin. In fact, one is more often concerned with excluding a tumor in the genitourinary tract than determining the exact etiology of hematuria. For this reason, an anatomic approach to the differential diagnosis of hematuria seems appropriate.

Etiology

The more common causes of hematuria are listed in Table 2-1. Bleeding may arise from the urethra, prostate, bladder, ureter, or kidney. Urethral hematuria may be related to acute urethritis of any cause (although less commonly with chlamydia) or to a structural abnormality (e.g., urethral diverticulum). Lesions in the urethra usually cause dysuria. A recent change in sexual partner or urethral trauma may be important historical information. Hematuria in the first part of the stream is usually from the urethra. Terminal hematuria suggests a bladder neck or prostate source, and hematuria throughout the urine stream suggests a bladder, ureteral, or renal source.

Acute or chronic prostatitis and prostatic tumors can occasionally cause gross or microscopic hematuria. Digital rectal examination can usually distinguish these, but cystourethroscopy may be necessary.

Bleeding from the urinary bladder is common with transitional cell carcinoma, interstitial cystitis, cystolithiasis or bacterial cystitis. In long-distance runners, trauma and inflammation of the bladder trigone can cause gross or microscopic hematuria. This and other causes of bladder hematuria are easily identifiable with cystoscopy.

A pyelogram (retrograde or antegrade) is usually necessary to

Table 2-1 Common Causes of Hematuria

Urethra
    Urethritis
    Diverticulum
    Carbuncle
    Trauma*
    Stones
    Malignancy
    Tuberculosis
    Extrinsic disease (tumors, abscess)

Prostate
    Acute prostatitis
    Chronic prostatitis
    Prostatic carcinoma
    Prostatic hyperplasia

Bladder
    Bacterial cystitis
    Interstitial cystitis
    Malignancy
    Stones
    Trauma*

Kidney
    Glomerular
      Asymptomatic ("benign hematuria")
          Benign familial hematuria
          Berger's (IgA) nephropathy
      Nephrotic syndrome
      Nephritic syndrome
      Rapidly progressive GN
      Chronic GN
    Nonglomerular
      Interstitial nephritis
      Papillary necrosis (analgesic, diabetic, sickle cell)
      Vascular disease (emboli, malignant hypertension, AV malformation)
    Cysts
    Malignancy
    Trauma*

---

*Includes procedures such as catheterization, cystoscopy, and percutaneous
    nephrostomy.

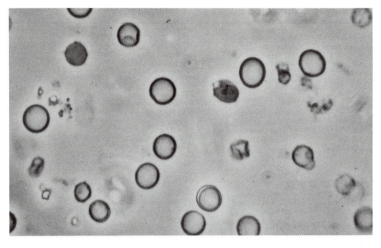

A

Figure 2-1: *A,* Urinary RBCs under phase microscopy from a patient with nonglomerular bleeding. Cells are isomorphic.

determine the cause of ureteral bleeding. Calculi and transitional cell carcinoma are the most common causes of ureteral bleeding.

Renal causes of hematuria can be glomerular or nonglomerular in origin. The RBC cast is virtually diagnostic of glomerular bleeding. In addition, a markedly distorted RBC surface is highly predictive of glomerular pathology (Fig. 2-1). RBC surface changes are most easily seen under phase microscopy. These "dysmorphic" RBCs are believed to arise from physical distortion of the RBC membrane induced by the wide variation in osmolarity (50 mOsm/L to 1,200 mOsm/L and pH (7.4 to 4.5) along the renal tubule. Concurrent 3+ or 4+ proteinuria by dipstick is suggestive (but not diagnostic) of glomerular hematuria. This should be confirmed by 24-hour quantitative collection and possibly electrophoresis.

Of the glomerular disorders (see Chapter 4), nephrotic syndrome, nephritic syndrome, rapidly progressive glomerulonephritis (GN), and chronic GN are all commonly associated with either

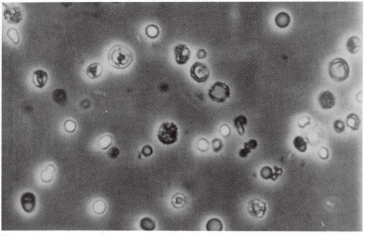

B

Figure 2-1: *B,* Urinary RBCs from a patient with a glomerular hematuria. Note the number of different sizes and shapes.

proteinuria, hypertension, or azotemia. Isolated hematuria of glomerular origin is generally benign, and may be "benign familial hematuria" (thin basement membrane disease) or a focal glomerulonephritis. The latter is most commonly caused by immunoglobulin A (IgA) nephropathy (Berger's disease) (see Chapter 4). The former may be a milder variant of familial nephritis. Nevertheless, without proteinuria, hypertension, or azotemia, isolated glomerular hematuria is usually a relatively benign condition for which there is no effective therapy. A renal biopsy is therefore not usually recommended in this setting.

Dysmorphic RBCs and RBC casts are generally not seen when renal bleeding is of nonglomerular origin. Vascular disease, interstitial nephritis, papillary necrosis, trauma, and tumors may all cause bleeding from the kidney. Cystoscopic observation of the ureteral orifices for hematuria is helpful in identifying unilateral causes of renal bleeding such as tumor, arteriovenous malformations, or embolus. Selective ureteral catheterization may be helpful, but ureteral catheter passage itself may cause hematuria in a normal upper urinary tract.

Diagnostic Approach

Based on these observations, one can develop a rational diagnostic approach to patients with hematuria (Fig. 2-2). First a positive dipstick or even "gross" hematuria must be confirmed by microscopic examination of the sediment. False-positive dipsticks can result from hemoglobinuria, myoglobinuria, or ascorbic acid and are very common with some of the commercially available dipsticks. Secondly, although most patients with hematuria have a urologic abnormality requiring cystoscopy and pyelography, patients with obvious glomerular disease or urinary infection can be selected on the basis of the urinary sediment. RBC casts or unequivocally dysmorphic RBCs by phase microscopy would sufficiently implicate glomerular disease such that cystoscopy and pyelography could be bypassed. Similarly, pyuria with dysuria, WBC casts, and bacteriuria are sufficient to initiate treatment for a urinary tract infection (pyelonephritis, cystitis, or urethritis). However, one must maintain a high degree of suspicion for urologic tumors and other anatomic abnormalities. Therefore, hematuria that fails to clear after adequate treatment for urinary infection or which is not definitely diagnosed as a glomerular process must be re-evaluated by urography and cystoscopy.

Unless patients demonstrate clear-cut signs of glomerular disease or infection, the urinary tract should be visualized by intravenous pyelography with voiding as well as postvoid films and cystoscopy. This should identify specific abnormalities of the urethra, prostate, bladder, and upper urinary tract and allow specific treatment for those processes. If no abnormality of these structures is found, renal hematuria must be reconsidered.

Finally, arteriography and/or CT scanning should be reserved for those patients with unilateral hematuria of unknown cause or for cases in which further anatomic definition of a lesion is required. Renal biopsy is reserved for the assessment of glomerular diseases (see Chapter 4).

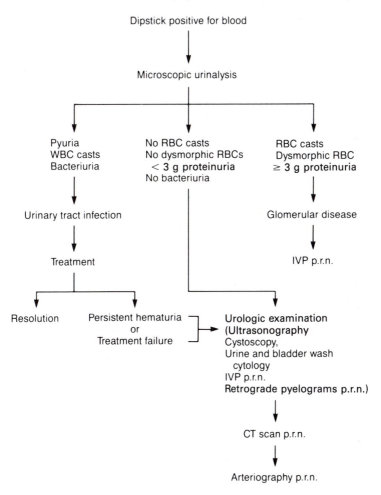

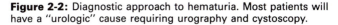

Figure 2-2: Diagnostic approach to hematuria. Most patients will have a "urologic" cause requiring urography and cystoscopy.

Proteinuria

Clinical disorders characterized by proteinuria may range from a mild, even transient, asymptomatic abnormality to a severe and unrelenting nephrotic syndrome. The diagnostic approach to patients with proteinuria is based on the normal physiology of renal protein–handling.

Urinary protein excretion depends on three major factors: (1) the physical characteristics and plasma concentration of protein, (2) the permeability of the glomerular capillary wall to protein, and (3) the tubular reabsorption of filtered protein (Fig. 2-3 and Table 2-2). Tubular secretion is not believed to play a major role in pathologic proteinuric states.

The ability of any protein to undergo filtration is dependent on the molecular size, shape, and charge of the protein. Filtration is enhanced as the molecular size decreases and the charge becomes more positive. Globulins of low molecular weight, usually positively charged, are therefore easily filterable. Any increase in their plasma concentration will usually result in increased urinary excretion (overflow proteinuria). Alternatively, albumin is larger and negatively charged and is filtered only minimally in the normal individual. The ability of albumin to undergo filtration is therefore dependent on glomerular permeability, not plasma concentration. Glomerular permeability is critically dependent on negatively charged sialoproteins, which are a structural component on the urinary side of the glomerular capillary wall. Loss of these negative charges (the glomerular membrane becoming more positively charged) or structural disruption of the glomerular basement mem-

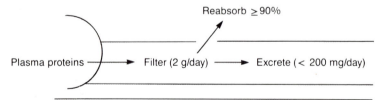

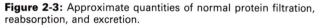

Figure 2-3: Approximate quantities of normal protein filtration, reabsorption, and excretion.

Table 2-2 Determinants of Normal Protein Filtration, Reabsorption, and Excretion

Plasma protein	Tubular reabsorption
Size	Protein size
Charge	Urine flow
Shape	Tubular cell function
Concentration	
Glomerular capillary wall	
Fixed negative charges	
Basement membrane structure	

brane allows filtration of the larger, negatively charged albumin (glomerular proteinuria).

In normal individuals, approximately 1 to 3 g of protein, most of which are small molecular globulins, are filtered every 24 hours. Ninety percent of filtered protein is reabsorbed by the renal tubules by active processes. Some of this reabsorbed protein is metabolized by the renal tubular cells; some is returned to the peritubular circulation. Any disease affecting the viability of the tubules or interstitium (tubulointerstitial nephritis) may decrease this physiologic protein reabsorption, resulting in greater protein excretion (tubulointerstitial proteinuria).

Overflow Proteinuria

Overflow proteinuria occurs when a normally filtered protein is overproduced in the plasma and "overflows" into the urine. The most striking example of this phenomenon is the multiple myeloma, where the paraprotein (Bence Jones protein) appears in the urine as a monoclonal ("M") spike. Another common example is myoglobinuria seen with rhabdomyolysis or after an acute myocardial infarction. On urinary protein electrophoresis, this appears as a slightly broader-based increase in gamma globulin. Lysozymuria seen in patients with myelogenous leukemia is another example of overflow proteinuria.

One must remember that chemical dipsticks used to detect urinary protein react with albumin only and that Bence Jones protein and other overflow proteinurias will be missed when dipstick testing alone is used. To detect urinary globulins, sulfosalicylic acid or heat acetic methods must be used. This is routinely performed by most hospital laboratories but rarely by "office labs." Thus, clinical suspicion of myeloma or myoglobinuria requires that one of these methods and/or electrophoresis be done.

Glomerular Proteinuria

A change in permeability of the glomerular filtration barrier will increase filtration once excretion of protein as the capacity to reabsorb is quickly superseded. Such *glomerular proteinuria* may result from a structural derangement of the glomerular basement membrane (e.g., diabetic nephropathy, membranous GN) or a loss of its fixed negative charges (e.g., minimal change GN). Although mild degrees of proteinuria can be seen, glomerular proteinuria is often massive (>3.5 g/1.73 m^2/day). If persistent, such "nephrotic range proteinuria" will eventually result in the hypoalbuminemia, edema, and hyperlipidemia known as the "nephrotic syndrome."

Typically, glomerular proteinuria includes the larger and more positively charged albumin, easily identified by electrophoresis. With more severe damage to the glomerular basement membrane (e.g., amyloidosis), all plasma proteins will readily appear in the urine and the urinary protein electrophoresis will mimic the serum.

Proteinuria of glomerular origin is often associated with other abnormalities such as hematuria (dysmorphic RBCs and/or RBC casts), nephrotic syndrome (proteinuria [>3.5 g/day], hypoalbuminemia, edema, and hyperlipidemia), hypertension and azotemia. The diagnostic approach to patients with glomerular disease is presented in Chapter 4.

Tubulointerstitial Proteinuria

The typical urinary electrophoretic pattern for tubulointerstitial nephritis is a broad polyclonal increase in the globulin region. Presumably this occurs because of tubular dysfunction and failure to reabsorb and/or metabolize normally filtered globulins. The inflammatory process may also cause secretion of protein into the urine, enhancing the globulin band. One should remember that any normally filtered protein may appear in the urine with tubulointerstitial nephritis. Light-chains, for example, may not necessarily indicate myeloma but may appear in a variety of interstitial nephritides. Urine immunoelectrophoresis may therefore be necessary to distinguish "free" light-chains (myeloma) in this setting.

Because tubulointerstitial proteinuria is caused largely by a failure of reabsorption of normally filtered proteins, there are typically 1 to 1.5 g of proteins in the urine daily and nearly always less than 2 g daily. However, as the tubulointerstitial disease progresses, the glomerulus is often damaged secondarily so that albuminuria and (rarely) nephrotic-range proteinuria can be seen. Therefore, during the late stages of tubulointerstitial nephritis, urinary protein electrophoresis is a less valuable diagnostic tool.

Transient or Temporary Proteinuria

Persistent proteinuria generally indicates significant renal parenchymal disease and requires further evaluation with 24-hour quantitation, urinary electrophoresis, and possibly renal biopsy. However, proteinuria may often be transient during the day or temporary, lasting only a few days. Transient or temporary proteinuria usually indicates a functional condition, usually reversible and rarely leading to significant renal disease.

Orthostatic proteinuria is one such functional syndrome. During their second or third decade of life, patients are usually discovered to have proteinuria on urinalysis. Interestingly, these individuals will excrete abnormal quantities of protein only when in an upright position; when supine, protein excretion is perfectly normal. Presumably this results from altered intrarenal hemodynamics that occur when the patient assumes an upright posture, but the precise pathophysiology is unknown. Long-term follow-up studies prove that orthostatic proteinuria is a benign condition not associated with renal function deterioration. Orthostatic proteinuria can be documented by sequential 12-hour urine collections with the patient in the upright and supine postures.

Transient or temporary proteinuria is also associated with several nonrenal disorders. These include sepsis, seizures, high fever, congestive heart failure, and pancreatitis. The cause of proteinuria in these cases is unknown and different mechanisms may be operative in different cases. Nevertheless, the proteinuria appears to be functional, resolving as the underlying condition resolves, usually within 3 to 5 days. Further evaluation of these patients is rarely warranted, although follow-up 3 to 6 months later is appropriate.

Diagnostic Approach

Figure 2-4 outlines our basic diagnostic approach to the patient with proteinuria. If dipstick testing is used to screen for proteinuria, false-negative tests must be considered. If Bence Jones proteinuria is suspected, a confirmatory test should be performed (sulfosalicyclic acid, heat acetic acid, electrophoresis).

Once proteinuria has been confirmed, one must consider functional proteinuria. Functional proteinuria is usually transient, resolving with improvement of the underlying medical condition (e.g., seizures, sepsis, fever). Orthostatic proteinuria can be excluded by a 24-hour urine collection divided into two approximately equal 12-hour collections, with the patient in the upright and recumbent positions, respectively. No further evaluation of functional proteinuria is necessary.

For the remainder of patients with persistent proteinuria, a thoughtful microscopic examination of the urinary sediment, a quantitative 24-hour urine collection for protein, and in many cases, urine protein electrophoresis should be performed. Based on their results, the proteinuria can be categorized as overflow, glomerular, or tubulointerstitial, allowing the clinician to generate an appropriate differential diagnosis.

Azotemia

Distinguishing acute from chronic azotemia is the first step in the evaluation of the patient with an elevated BUN or creatinine. A variety of tests are helpful in this regard (Table 2-3) including the

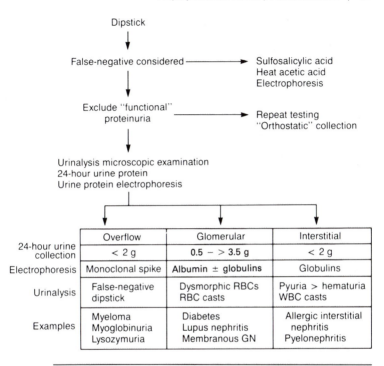

Figure 2-4: Diagnostic approach to patients with proteinuria.

history (from the patient or medical record), the rate of rise of creatinine, renal size, and serum albumin, and the hematocrit. Although none of these tests approaches 100% accuracy, taken together, they will usually result in the correct diagnosis.

The clinical history is probably the most important of these differentiating tests. The patient may know of previously abnormal kidney tests, hypertension, urinary infection, proteinuria, or hematuria. If available, previous hospital or office medical records can be invaluable. A family history of known kidney disease or early death might indicate a chronic renal disease. In addition, the recent onset

Table 2-3 Aids in Distinguishing Acute Azotemia From Chronic Azotemia

	Acute	*Chronic*
Previous tests	Normal	Azotemia
Family history	Negative	May be positive
Symptoms	Abrupt	Indolent
Rate of serum creatinine rise	Daily	Monthly
Laboratory		
Hematocrit	Normal	Low
Serum albumin	Normal	Normal to slightly low
Imaging		
Renal size	Normal to large	Usually small
Echogenicity	Lucent	Dense

of symptoms, either uremic or related to an acute illness, would suggest a more acute process.

If the above historic information is unobtainable or is inconclusive, other tests may be helpful. The rate of serum creatinine rise is usually rapid in acute renal failure, typically 0.5 to 1.5 mg/dl/day. Hypoalbuminemia or significant anemia would suggest a more chronic process. Similarly, radiographs revealing small kidneys and increased echogenicity by ultrasonography support a more chronic process. These latter tests are also useful in predicting potential reversibility.

(The differential diagnosis and approach to acute azotemia are extensively outlined in Chapter 3 and will not be discussed further here.)

Diagnostic Approach

Once a chronic process has been established, the clinician should consider whether the disorder affects primarily the renal glomerulus (glomerulonephritis), tubules and interstitium (interstitial nephritis), or blood vessels. This may be difficult, particularly when the disease has been present for many years. Nevertheless, distinguishing between glomerular, interstitial, or vascular processes should enable the clinician to generate a more complete differential diagnosis.

Several tests help one make this distinction (Table 2-4). Of these, evaluation of the urinary protein excretion is best. Patients with nephrotic-range proteinuria (excreting >3.5 g of protein per day) are considered to have glomerular disease. Although patients with primary interstitial processes may sometimes present with this degree of proteinuria, excretion of much less urinary protein (gener-

Table 2-4 Tests Used in the Differential Diagnosis of Chronic Azotemia

Test	Glomerular	Interstitial	Vascular
Urinary protein (g/24h)	≥3.5 g	<2 g	Variable
Qualitative	Albumin > globulin	Globulin >> albumin	Albumin and globulins
Urinalysis-sediment	"Active" Dysmorphic RBCs Granular casts RBC casts	"Bland" Pyuria > hematuria Occasional WBC casts	Hematuria Pyuria "Telescoped"
Hyperkalemia	Seen at end-stage renal disease	Out of proportion to GFR	With end-stage renal disease
Acidosis	High anion gap. Seen at end-stage renal disease	Hyperchloremic Before end-stage renal disease	With end-stage renal disease
Hypertension	3–4 +	1–2 +	3–4 +
IVP	Variable size Smooth surface	Small kidneys May have irregular cortical scarring Clubbed calyces	Small Usually smooth surface Calyces normal
Uric acid (serum)	Normal	Often high	Normal

ally <1.5 g/day) is more typical. In addition, albuminuria generally indicates glomerulopathy, whereas urinary globulins are usually seen with interstitial nephritis. Therefore, electrophoresis of the urine may be a helpful diagnostic test. However, the more chronic the disease process, the less helpful the urine protein electrophoresis. Because there is usually both glomerular and interstitial damage with vascular disease, the quantitative urinary protein and electrophoresis is variable. Generally both albumin and globulins are excreted in the non-nephrotic range.

The urinary sediment is typically bland with chronic interstitial nephritis, regardless of the etiology. Glomerulonephritis usually presents a more active sediment with RBCs (usually dysmorphic), granular casts, and occasionally, RBC casts. The urinary sediment in chronic vascular disease may mimic either chronic interstitial nephritis or glomerulonephritis. The simultaneous occurrence of proteinuria, RBC casts, and WBC casts ("telescoped" urine sediment) strongly suggests vascular disease.

Because urinary potassium and acid excretion are dependent on tubular secretion of potassium and hydrogen ion, hyperkalemia and metabolic acidosis are more commonly seen with interstitial nephritis. The hyperkalemia usually appears long before the glomerular filtration rate falls to critically low levels. The metabolic acidosis is usually of the hyperchloremic non-anion gap variety, indicating that uremic acids (phosphates and sulfates) have not yet accumulated. Both the hyperkalemia and metabolic acidosis of interstitial nephropathies can be seen with a relatively good glomerular filtration rate (C_{cr} >10 ml/min). Hyperkalemia and hyperchloremic acidosis are less common with vascular diseases.

Less reliable clues of interstitial nephritis are anemia (out of proportion to the GFR) and hyperuricemia. Hypertension is slightly more typical with glomerular or vascular disease.

Because the kidney has a limited capacity to respond to injury, any primary disease process (glomerular, interstitial, or vascular) can effect changes on other structures. For example, severe glomerular changes such as focal and segmental sclerosis are typically seen with progression of primarily interstitial diseases such as analgesic nephropathy or pyelonephritis caused by vesicoureteral reflux. Similarly, glomerulopathies, such as Alport's syndrome (hereditary nephritis) or membranoproliferative glomerulonephritis commonly cause intense tubulointerstitial scarring and fibrosis. The interstitial changes are so impressive with hereditary nephritis that it is often classified as an interstitial nephritis. Thus, as any renal disease progresses toward end-stage, its clinical and histologic manifestations become indistinct and clear classification as a primary glomerular, tubulointerstitial, or vascular process becomes impossible. A general diagnostic approach to patients with isolated azotemia is shown in Figure 2-5.

Often, an acute deterioration in renal function may occur in patients with pre-existing renal disease—i.e., *acute on chronic azotemia*. For example, Figure 2-6 illustrates the case of a patient with slowly progressive azotemia (e.g., caused by chronic glomerulonephritis) whose renal function acutely exacerbates, deviating

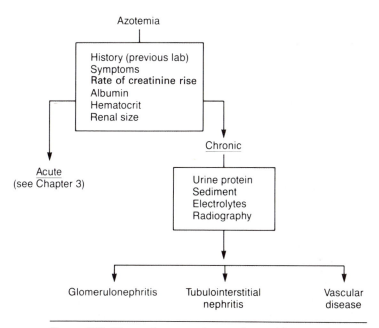

Figure 2-5: Diagnostic approach to patients with azotemia.

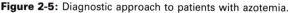

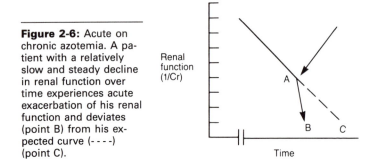

Figure 2-6: Acute on chronic azotemia. A patient with a relatively slow and steady decline in renal function over time experiences acute exacerbation of his renal function and deviates (point B) from his expected curve (- - - -) (point C).

significantly from the expected curve for his disease. There are a variety of causes for such an exacerbation, most of which are readily reversible. Thus, it behooves the clinician to search diligently for these potentially reversible factors.

An acronym that outlines the possible causes of acute on chronic azotemia is "FIASCO":

F = Fluid (congestive failure or volume depletion)

I = Infection (urinary tract or systemic)

A = Arteriovenous (hypertension, thrombosis, embolus, venous thrombosis)

S = Substances (drugs, radiographic contrast)

C = Consumption (excessive dietary protein or phosphorus)

O = Obstruction

Hypertension

The first and most important diagnostic step when treating patients with hypertension is to distinguish the small percentage of patients with a secondary cause from the majority with primary or essential hypertension. The common causes of secondary hypertension are listed in Table 2-5 and catalogued clinically in Table 2-6.

Table 2-5 Common Causes of Secondary Hypertension

Renal artery stenosis
  Atherosclerotic
  Fibromuscular

Renal parenchymal disease
  Glomerulonephritis
  Diabetic nephropathy
  Polycystic kidney
  Obstruction

Adrenal cortex
  Cushing's syndrome (hyperplasia)
  Conn's syndrome (adenoma)

Pheochromocytoma

Coarctation of the aorta

Renal Artery Stenosis

Renal artery stenosis (RAS) most commonly occurs as a result of atherosclerotic occlusion of the renal arteries in patients older than 50 years of age with generalized atherosclerosis. In younger patients (usually women) it may arise from fibromuscular hyperplasia of the renal arteries. The resultant hypertension is usually severe, labile, and often is resistant to therapy. If it is unilateral, the patients are usually volume-contracted (because of overperfusion and diuresis in the contralateral kidney) and often have orthostatic hypotension. When the stenosis is bilateral, however, volume expansion is the rule. Thus, unilateral renal artery stenosis causes high plasma renin activity, whereas bilateral stenosis causes a volume-mediated hypertension with normal plasma renin.

An abdominal bruit is present in as many as 70% of patients with RAS, but is also present in 10 to 30% of those with essential hypertension. Because there are many more patients with essential hypertension than RAS, most patients with a renal or abdominal bruit do not have RAS. Thus, neither an abdominal bruit nor plasma renin level are sensitive or specific enough to distinguish RAS from essential hypertension.

Similarly, the common radiographs (hypertensive IVP, nuclear

Table 2-6 Typical Historical, Physical, and Laboratory Features of the Common Causes of Secondary Hypertension

Cause	History	Examination	Findings Lab	Diagnostic Test
RAS	Abrupt onset Age <30, >50 Severe, labile	Abdominal bruit Postural hypotension (unilateral) Edema (bilateral)	Hypokalemic alkalosis	IVP (screening) Arteriogram (anatomic) Captopril test (functional)
RPD	Renal disease	Pallor	Azotemia Proteinuria Hematuria	IVP
Adrenal Cushing's syndrome	Glucose intolerance	Central obesity Striae Hirsutism	Hypokalemic alkalosis Hyperglycemia	Excess plasma cortisol after dexa- methasone
Conn's syndrome	Polyuria, polydipsia	Edema	Hypokalemic alkalosis	Low plasma renin High plasma aldosterone
Pheochromocytoma	Palpitation Perspiration Paroxysms	Postural hypotension		Urinary norepinephrine Plasma norepinephrine after clonidine
Coarctation	Lower extremity weakness Claudication	Decreased leg blood pressure Delayed femoral pulse		Arteriogram

If any of these factors are identified on the initial evaluation of hypertension, the appropriate diagnostic tests can be pursued.

scan, and even intravenous digital subtraction angiography) lack the sensitivity or specificity to identify RAS consistently. IVP however, does allow evaluation of possible ureteral obstruction and other renal parenchymal diseases. Thus, despite its shortcomings, the IVP remains the best radiograph for evaluating the possibility of secondary hypertension. When screening for RAS, however, one must rely on a strong clinical suspicion and a combination of findings (e.g., an abdominal bruit, high plasma renin, and compatible IVP).

The most sensitive and specific radiograph is selective renal arteriography and the clinician should not hesitate to perform this test early if the clinical suspicion of RAS is high. In patients older than 50 years of age, however, renal artery stenosis may be anatomically present but functionally insignificant. In this patient population, renal vein renin sampling (demonstrating ipsilateral hypersecretion and contralateral suppression) or a "captopril test" (demonstrating an abrupt increase from baseline in peripheral or renal vein renin 1 hour after the administration of oral captopril) will therefore define functionally significant RAS. Nuclear blood flow scans before and after administration of captopril are similarly useful (Fig. 2-7) A diagnostic approach to the patient with renal artery stenosis is outlined in Figure 2-8.

Renal Parenchymal Disease

A variety of *renal parenchymal diseases* (RPD) may cause hypertension. Glomerular disease (in particular diabetes and the nephritic syndromes), polycystic kidney disease, and obstructive uropathy are most typical. Hematuria, proteinuria, and/or azotemia are usually evident and serve as appropriate screening tests. An IVP (or renal ultrasonography if serum creatinine > 2 mg/dl) is the best initial imaging study.

Adrenal Cortex

Adrenal causes of secondary hypertension can be suspected if the electrolytes show hypokalemic metabolic alkalosis. *Cushing's syndrome* also produces physical findings of temporal

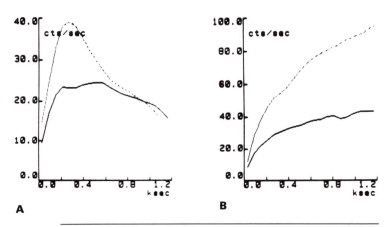

Figure 2-7: *A*, Renal hippuran nuclear scan in a patient with bilateral renal artery stenosis. This precaptopril scan suggests only unilateral stenosis. *B*, Postcaptopril hippuran in same patient shows significant alteration of both curves, indicating bilateral renal artery stenosis.

balding, centripetal obesity, abdominal striae, and hirsutism. The diagnosis rests on demonstrating nonsuppressible plasma cortisol after dexamethasone administration. *Conn's syndrome* (primary hyperaldosteronism) often produces slight edema (see Chapter 7), and polyuria with polydipsia is not uncommon. If suspected, a low plasma renin, high plasma aldosterone level, and adrenal mass as determined by CT scanning confirms the diagnosis.

Pheochromocytoma

The typical history of a patient with *pheochromocytoma* is paroxysms of hypertension with flushing, palpitation, perspiration, headache, and weight loss. Postural hypotension is usually evident. Twenty-four-hour urinary norepinephrine and an elevated plasma norepinephrine (pheochromocytoma not suppressed by oral clonidine) are the best diagnostic tests. The tumors are usually located in the adrenal glands (in 90% of patients) or along the thoracic and abdominal spine.

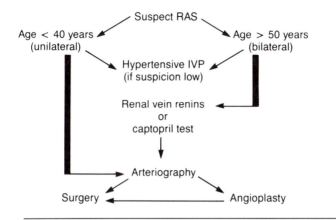

Figure 2-8: A diagnostic approach to RAS suspected from the history, physical examination, and initial laboratory screening of hypertensive patients. If the clinical suspicion is strong in young patients likely to have unilateral disease, an early arteriogram is indicated. If the clinical suspicion is low, a negative IVP will usually exclude the diagnosis. In patients older than 50 years of age, who are more likely to have bilateral or functionally insignificant disease, renal vein renin sampling or a "captopril" test should be done before or in conjunction with arteriography.

From the description of the common causes of secondary hypertension given in Table 2-6, one can develop a list of historical, physical, and laboratory clues that would prompt further evaluation. Ordinarily an initial history, physical examination, urinalysis, and chemistry profile will suffice. However, if one identifies any features suggestive of secondary hypertension, the diagnostic tests outlined in Table 2-6 can be pursued.

Case 2-1: *Discussion*

1. The presence of dysmorphic RBCs in the urine sediment of this patient strongly suggests glomerulonephritis. This could be confirmed if RBC casts are also identified.

2. The history is most consistent with IgA nephropathy (Berger's disease). With Berger's disease, the hematuria accompanies a febrile illness, whereas a postinfectious (e.g., poststreptococcal) glomerulonephritis would cause hematuria 2 to 4 weeks after the infection. Another possibility is benign familial hematuria (thin basement membrane disease). Other more aggressive causes of glomerular hematuria such as systemic lupus erythematosus (SLE), hereditary nephritis, and vasculitis should be excluded by appropriate testing (see Chapter 4). If these are excluded and the patient does not have proteinuria, azotemia, or hypertension, a renal biopsy, although diagnostic, is usually unnecessary. The patient should be followed at 6-month intervals with close attention to urine sediment, proteinuria, blood pressure, and renal function. If these are abnormal, a renal biopsy is indicated.

IVP is probably unnecessary in this patient. Cystoscopy is not necessary.

Case 2-2: *Discussion*

In the absence of urinary tract infection symptoms, pyuria, bacteriuria, dysmorphic RBCs, RBC casts and significant proteinuria, the most likely cause of the hematuria is a structural abnormality of the urinary tract (Fig. 2-2). Because the hematuria is throughout the urinary stream, its source is probably in the urinary bladder, ureters, or kidneys. In this age group, the major concern is a genitourinary neoplasm.

As the first diagnostic step, IVP with nephrotomograms should be used. In this patient's case, these showed normal kidneys and ureters. There was a filling defect at the base of the bladder consistent with the patient's prior transurethral prostatectomy, and there was a 1.5- by 1.0-cm filling defect in the left lateral superior aspect of the bladder which was best seen on the postvoid film. Because of the bladder filling defect, the patient had cystoscopy with anesthesia that revealed a papillary tumor. This was resected under the same anesthetic and was a Grade II transitional cell carcinoma.

Case 2-3: *Discussion*

In this patient with persistent proteinuria, a 24-hour urine collection divided into two 12-hour collections (with the patient in the upright and supine positions, respectively) should be performed. In her case, the results were a urine protein of 648 mg (upright) and 423 mg (supine), thus excluding the possibility of orthostatic proteinuria.

In order to exclude overflow proteinuria and distinguish between glomerular and interstitial disease, a urine protein electrophoresis should be ordered. This showed albumin in the urine almost exclusively, suggesting glomerular disease. Repeated close examinations of the urine sediment showed several RBCs with dysmorphic changes, again suggestive of glomerular disease.

A renal biopsy should then be performed to define glomerular histology. The biopsy showed a mild mesangial proliferative glomerulonephritis with immunoglobulin G(IgG), A(IgA), and C3 deposits in capillary loops. Electron microscopy revealed focal subepithelial dense deposits. The renal biopsy was believed to be consistent with lupus nephropathy. A repeat ANA was indeed positive at 1:2560. In this case, the urine protein electrophoresis and microscopic sediment examination help identify the renal parenchymal process as glomerular.

Case 2-4: *Discussion*

1. Anemia and the relative lack of symptoms point to *chronic* azotemia.

2. Low serum albumin, previous laboratory values showing azotemia and small (<9 cm) echogenic kidneys confirm that the process is chronic. An IVP would not be helpful here. This degree of azotemia precludes good visualization and increases the risk of contrast toxicity.

3. Chronic *interstitial* nephritis is suggested by (1) a bland urinary sediment with a predominance of pyuria, (2) the hyperchloremic (non-anion gap) acidosis with hyperkalemia despite a relatively well-preserved GFR (C_{cr} of 20 ml/minute), and (3) minimal proteinuria. In view of this patient's chronic pain syndrome (headaches) and previous ulcer disease, analgesic nephropathy is the most likely etiology of her renal disease.

Case 2-5: *Discussion*

1. The long duration and positive family history of hypertension in this woman suggest primary or essential hypertension. However, the hypokalemia (2.8 mEq/L) and metabolic alkalosis (HCO_3 = 30 mEq/L) are suggestive of renal artery stenosis (with secondary hyperaldosteronism) or a primary adrenal gland problem (Cushing's or Conn's syndrome). Although hypokalemic alkalosis is usually caused by diuretic administration, the patient reported taking no medicines for the past year. Therefore, further evaluation to exclude mineralocorticoid excess is needed.

2. The lack of orthostatic hypotension and the presence of edema also suggest an adrenal problem (although bilateral renal artery stenosis is usually a volume-expanded state without orthostatic hypotension). Testing with a plasma cortisol after administration of 1 mg dexamethasone was found to be normal, effectively excluding Cushing's syndrome. However, plasma renin level was low (<1 pg/ml) and did not rise after administration of furosemide. In addition, her plasma aldosterone level was high. CT scanning confirmed the presence of a small right adrenal mass. Histology on the lesion revealed a primary adrenal adenoma.

References

Abuelo JG. Proteinuria: diagnostic principles and procedures. Ann Int Med 1983; 98:186–191.

Corwin HL, Silverstein MD. The diagnosis of neoplasia in patients with asymptomatic microscopic hematuria: a decision analysis. J Urol 1988; 139:1002–1006.

Fairley KF, Birch DF. Hematuria: a simple method for identifying glomerular bleeding. Kidney Int 1982; 21:105–108.

Geyskes GG, Oei HY, Puylaert C, Mers E. Renovascular hypertension identified by captopril-induced changes in the renogram. Hypertension 1987; 9:451–458.

Kristal B, Shasha SM, Labin L, Cohen A. Estimation of quantitative proteinuria by using the protein-creatinine ratio in random urine samples. Am J Nephrol 1988; 8:198–203.

Muller FB, Sealey JE, Case DB, et al. The captopril test for identifying renovascular disease in hypertensive patients. Am J Med 1986; 80:633–644.

Raman GV, Pead L, Lee HA, Maskell R. A blind controlled trial of phase-contrast microscopy by two observers for evaluating the source of hematuria. Nephron 1986; 44:304–308.

Vaughan ED. Renovascular hypertension. Kidney Int 1985; 27:811–827.

Working Group on Renovascular Hypertension. Detection, evaluation and treatment of renovascular hypertension. Arch Int Med 1987; 147:820–829.

3   Acute Renal Failure

- Case Presentations

- Nonrenal Causes of Acute Azotemia

- Acute Renal Failure Versus Prerenal Azotemia

- Diagnostic Approach to Acute Azotemia

- Causes of Acute Renal Failure

- Diagnostic Approach to Acute Renal Failure

- Prevention of Acute Renal Failure

- Treatment and Prognosis of Acute Renal Failure

- Case Discussions

Case 3-1

A previously well 46-year-old man was admitted with acute pulmonary edema and an acute myocardial infarction. He was treated with furosemide and improved. On Day 10, he was noted to have a BUN of 100 mg/dl and creatinine level of 4.2 mg/dl. The following table shows the results of laboratory tests.

	Day 1	Day 10
BUN	10 mg/dl	100 mg/dl
Creatinine	1.0 mg/dl	4.2 mg/dl
Na	140 mEq/L	136 mEq/L
K	4.4 mEq/L	3.2 mEq/L
Cl	102 mEq/L	94 mEq/L
HCO₃	26 mEq/L	32 mEq/L
Weight	72 kg	67 kg

Questions

1. What are the possible diagnoses to explain the patient's azotemia?
2. What further diagnostic tests should be performed?
3. Do the electrolytes suggest a cause for the azotemia?

Case 3-2

A 72-year-old man was admitted because of extreme lethargy and confusion. One week before admission, he had complained of cold symptoms and took an antihistamine preparation. The following table shows the results of laboratory tests.

BUN	244 mg/dl
Creatinine	19 mg/dl
Na	142 mEq/L
K	5.6 mEq/L
Cl	112 mEq/L
HCO₃	18 mEq/L
Hgb/Hct	14.8/45
Urinalysis	Difficult to obtain

Questions

1. Does the patient have acute or chronic azotemia?
2. What are the possible diagnoses?
3. What is the next diagnostic/therapeutic step?

Case 3-3

A 43-year-old woman was admitted for calf claudication. She was an insulin-dependent diabetic and had been for 12 years. On Day 2 of her hospital stay, she underwent arteriography for peripheral vascular disease. She was asymptomatic throughout her stay at the hospital. The following table shows the results of laboratory tests on Days 1 through 8.

	Day 1	Day 2	Day 4	Day 8
BUN	18 mg/dl	19 mg/dl	64 mg/dl	44 mg/dl
Creatinine	2.0 mg/dl	1.9 mg/dl	5.2 mg/dl	4.1 mg/dl
Na	140 mEq/L		140 mEq/L	140 mEq/L
K	5.2 mEq/L		6.2 mEq/L	6.2 mEq/L
Cl	112 mEq/L		114 mEq/L	115 mEq/L
HCO₃	18 mEq/L		16 mEq/L	15 mEq/L
Glucose	368 mg/dl		280 mg/dl	220 mg/dl
Urinalysis (protein)	4+ (protein)			
Urine output			1500 ml/day	

Questions

1. Why did the patient become azotemic on Day 4?
2. What may be done to prevent this complication?
3. What was done between Days 4 and 8 to improve the situation?
4. What is the cause of this patient's azotemia and proteinuria?
5. What is the likely cause of her electrolyte picture on admission?

Case 3-4

A 64-year-old man was admitted for abdominal pain. Temperature was 103°F. The WBC count is 24,600 with 84 segmented neutrophils (segs) and 14 bands. Abdominal examination and radiographs suggested acute mechanical small bowel obstruction. On the following day, a ruptured sigmoid colon diverticulum was surgically treated. The following table shows the results of laboratory tests.

You are asked to see the patient on the 1st postoperative day for oliguria.

	Admission	Day of Surgery	Postoperative Day 1
BUN	28 mg/dl	38 mg/dl	47 mg/dl
Creatinine	1.4 mg/dl	2.2 mg/dl	3.0 mg/dl
Urine output	300 ml/8 hr	450 ml/24 hrs	50 ml/8 hr
Weight	72 kg	78 kg	79 kg
Na	142 mEq/L		140 mEq/L
K	4.6 mEq/L		5 mEq/L
Cl	104 mEq/L		102 mEq/L
HCO₃	14 mEq/L		18 mEq/L
Hgb/Hct	14/42	9.8/29	9.6/28
Temperature	103°F	102.6°F	104°F
WBC	24,600	22,000	30,000

Questions

1. What is the cause of the patient's azotemia?
2. What further tests would you order on Day 3 to confirm your suspicion?
3. What is the cause of his metabolic acidosis?

Case 3-5

A 65-year-old man was admitted to the hospital with severe azotemia (BUN of 118 mg/dl; creatinine level of 7.9 mg/dl).

Two months earlier he presented with diffuse lymphadenopathy. At that time, his BUN was 27 and his creatinine was 1.2 mg/dl. Lymph node biopsy yielded a diagnosis of null cell, poorly differentiated lymphoma. His past history revealed that he was an insulin-dependent diabetic and was an occasionally steroid-dependent chronic asthmatic. His only medications were insulin and inhaled beclomethasone. He had received no chemotherapy.

Physical examination showed normal vital signs and slight expansion of extracellular fluid volume. Laboratory tests revealed a WBC of 7.6 with normal differential, hemoglobin level of 10.5 g/dl, and a platelet count of 313,000. Urinalysis showed granular casts, four to six WBC/hpf, 40 to 60 RBC/hpf, SG of 1.019, and 3 + proteinuria. Uric acid is 7.7 mg/dl, and phosphorus is 5.5 mg/dl. Liver function tests were normal. Creatine phosphokinase (CPK) was 44 mg/dl. Urine sodium was 61 mEq/L; FE_{NA} was 1.1%. Urine volume was 1,600 ml/day.

Over the next few days, BUN and creatinine continued to rise and dialysis was initiated.

Questions

1. What is the cause of the patient's acute azotemia?

Case 3-6

A 58-year-old man was admitted to the hospital because he had not urinated for 24 hours. He was taking no medications, and his review of systems was negative for cardiac, gastrointestinal, and genitourinary diseases. Vital signs were normal and there was no decrease in orthostatic blood pressure. Neck veins were not distended, there was no pedal edema, and the lungs and heart were normal to percussion and auscultation. Abdominal examination revealed no masses. Digital rectal examination revealed a hard, irregularly nodular prostate with extension into the pelvic side wall on the right. A 16-Fr Foley catheter was passed with ease into the bladder, revealing 50 ml of urine. Urinalysis shows a pH of 6, 1 + protein, no sugar, no bilirubin, trace blood, negative leukocyte esterase, negative nitrites, zero to two RBC/hpf, three WBC/hpf, and no bacteria. BUN was 96 mg/dl, serum creatinine was 13 mg/dl, WBC was 3.8, and hematocrit was 31%.

Questions

1. What other diagnostic steps should be taken?
2. What is the most likely diagnosis?

Acute azotemia is the most frequent nephrologic challenge. Acute azotemia may be caused by laboratory artifact, decreased renal perfusion (prerenal azotemia), or obstructive uropathy (postrenal azotemia). Acute renal failure (ARF), however, is defined as acute azotemia caused by renal disease only, and excludes pre- and postrenal factors. An increasing number of reports have documented ARF in nonoliguric patients, so that oliguria, once a hallmark of the syndrome, is no longer part of its definition.

The exclusion of pre- and postrenal causes of azotemia is crucial when evaluating patients with acute azotemia. Although the mortality rate for patients with ARF may be greater than 50%, pre- and postrenal azotemia are usually completely reversible. Because both pre- and postrenal azotemia can progress to established ARF if they are left unchecked, exclusion of such cases is mandatory.

Nonrenal Causes of Acute Azotemia

Artifact

Before an evaluation of any patient is made, the possibility of nonrenal factors affecting urea or creatinine should be considered (Table 3-1). Urea tends to increase whenever nitrogen substrate for urea production is increased. Protein breakdown from tissue catabolism, corticosteroids, gastrointestinal bleeding, or hyperalimentation can therefore markedly increase blood urea. Of course, intravascular volume contraction will increase urea by proximal tubular absorption (prerenal azotemia). On the other hand, hepatocellular failure, low protein intake, and volume excess are all associated with low BUN.

Serum creatinine may be increased by overproduction, blocked tubular secretion, or chemical interference with the serum creatinine (Jaffé) assay. Overproduction of creatinine most often occurs with rhabdomyolysis. Serum creatinine levels may be spuriously low in patients with cirrhosis, not only because of a decrease in muscle mass but also because of decreased conversion of creatine to creatinine in the liver.

Approximately 10 to 20% of excreted creatinine results from tubular secretion. Drugs competing with this secretion will increase serum creatinine independent of the glomerular filtration rate. Trimethoprim (Bactrim, Septra) and cimetidine (Tagamet) are two common drugs that elevate the serum creatinine by this mechanism.

Table 3-1 Nonrenal Factors Altering Urea or Creatinine

	Increased	*Decreased*
Urea	Prerenal azotemia Upper gastrointestinal bleeding Severe catabolic state Corticosteroids Hyperalimentation Tetracyclines	Hepatocellular failure Low protein intake Water excess (SIADH)

Creatinine	Overproduction
	  Rhabdomyolysis
	Blocked secretion
	  Trimethoprim
	  Cimetidine
	Chemical interference
	  Cefoxitin
	  Ascorbic acid
	  Acetone
	  Alphamethyldopa
		Decreased muscle mass
		
		Hepatocellular failure

SIADH = syndrome of inappropriate antidiuretic hormone.

In addition, chemicals may react as a noncreatinine chromogen in the Jaffé reaction—i.e., they are measured as creatinine. Cefoxitin, ascorbic acid, alpha methyldopa, and acetone can all spuriously raise the serum creatinine level. This chemical artifact explains the inordinant rise in the serum creatinine level in patients with ketoacidosis. The possibility of a spurious cause for azotemia should be considered early in the diagnostic approach to acute azotemia.

Postrenal Azotemia

If a patient has two functioning kidneys, a Foley catheter excludes obstructive uropathy of the bladder outlet. However, solitary kidneys are present in 1% of the general population and "functionally" solitary kidneys (i.e., where one kidney is nonfunctional) are even more common. Therefore, all patients with acute azotemia should undergo imaging of the urinary tract. Ultrasonography (Fig. 3-1) or CT scanning (without contrast) (Fig. 3-2) are safe and effective means of excluding obstructive uropathy in patients with two kidneys. If the ultrasonography or CT results are equivocal, a retrograde pyelogram to exclude obstructive uropathy should be considered.

Nuclear scanning, particularly with ^{131}I Hippuran, can also document obstruction by demonstrating the gradual and progressive accumulation of isotope with time. Although Hippuran scanning is

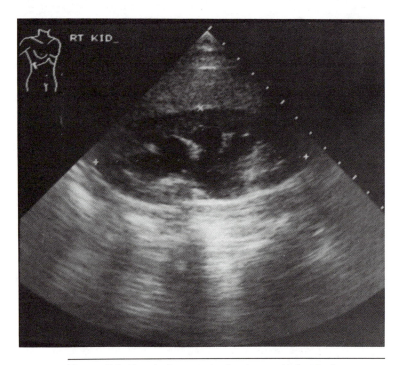

Figure 3-1: Renal ultrasonography demonstrating hydronephrosis in a patient with acute azotemia.

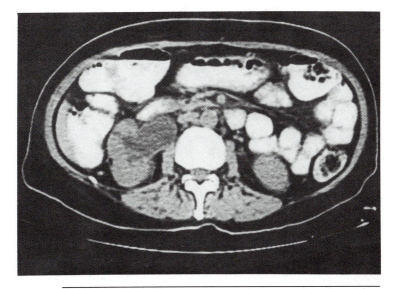

Figure 3-2: Noncontrast CT scan in patient with obstructive uropathy and acute azotemia.

less sensitive and specific than other studies for evaluating obstruction, it is also beneficial in evaluating tubular cell viability.

Whereas patients with ARF may be nonoliguric, patients with pre- and postrenal azotemia are usually oliguric (<500 mg of urine secreted per day). Exceptions to this rule are patients recently reported to have received drugs causing increased urine volume despite intravascular volume depletion (nonoliguric prerenal azotemia). Other exceptions include patients with partial urinary obstruction, where slight variation in daily output is common. Anuria (<50 ml of urine secreted per day) is usually seen only with complete urinary obstruction or severe compromise of renal circulation and cortical necrosis.

The common causes of postrenal azotemia are outlined in Table 3-2.

Table 3-2 Causes of Postrenal Azotemia

Lower urinary obstruction
   Urethral stricture
   Benign prostatic hypertrophy
   Prostatic carcinoma
   Bladder stone
   Bladder neck contracture

Upper urinary obstruction (bilateral or unilateral with only one
    kidney)
   Renal or ureteral stone
   Retroperitoneal fibrosis
   Malignancy of retroperitoneum or pelvic organs
   Ureteral tumor

Neurogenic bladder
   Diabetes mellitus
   Anticholinergic drugs
   Neurologic disorders

Prerenal Azotemia

The causes of prerenal azotemia are outlined in Table 3-3. The typical patient shows orthostatic hypotension, tachycardia, flat neck veins in the supine position, dry mucous membranes, and the other physical findings of extracellular volume (ECV) depletion (see Chapter 7). Peripheral and/or sacral edema, ascites, pulmonary rales, and jugular venous distention are absent in these patients. However, prerenal azotemia can also occur in patients with physical findings of ECV overload if the patient has a low "effective" circulating volume or if fluid is sequestered in a "third space" at the expense of the intravascular volume. Congestive heart failure is the most common example of the former. "Third space" losses are often a cause of acute azotemia in the postoperative setting.

Prerenal azotemia is a potentially reversible condition which if unrecognized may cause ARF in some patients. It is also the most common risk factor, predisposing to ARF. *The clinician should therefore make the exclusion of prerenal azotemia a prerequisite for the diagnosis of ARF.* If any doubt exists about the ECV status of a patient, early direct measurement of the pulmonary artery wedge pressure via Swan Ganz catheterization is recommended.

Table 3-3 Causes of Prerenal Azotemia

Low intravascular volume
  Hemorrhage
  Gastrointestinal losses
    Diarrhea
    Prolonged vomiting
    Enterocutaneous fistula or ileostomy
  Renal losses
    Diuretics
    Osmotic diuresis (hyperglycemia)

Low "effective" intravascular volume
  Poor cardiac output
  Ascites/cirrhosis
  Nephrotic syndrome

"Third space" losses
  Ascites
  Pancreatitis
  Peritonitis
  Hypoalbuminemia
  Abdominal surgery

Acute Renal Failure Versus Prerenal Azotemia

Before considering the etiologies of ARF, one must exclude the other common causes of acute azotemia. Artifacts are easily excluded by the history. A Foley catheter and renal ultrasonography exclude postrenal azotemia in most cases. The clinician is then left with the often difficult dilemma of differentiating prerenal azotemia from established ARF. As mentioned, the distinction is more than academic and one on which both treatment and prognosis hinge.

To exclude prerenal azotemia, a physical examination with careful attention to volume status is mandatory. In addition, thoughtful examination of the urinary sediment is often quite rewarding, sometimes resulting in the correct diagnosis.

The urinary sediment in patients with acute prerenal azotemia is usually bland. Because the urine is concentrated, low-grade proteinuria and occasionally granular casts can be seen. In sharp contrast is the urine sediment of a patient with ARF. Fine and coarse granular casts are typical, as are free red and white blood cells. Renal tubular epithelial cells, round and slightly larger than WBCs and with a central nucleus, are indicative of acute tubular necrosis (ATN) particularly when seen in large numbers. RBC casts and "dysmorphic" red cells are indicative of glomerulonephritis. Pyuria without bacteriuria, eosinophils (best identified by Hansel's stain) and WBC casts implicate interstitial nephritis as the cause of ARF. When all components (proteinuria, RBC and WBC casts, granular casts) are evident (the so-called "telescoped" urinary sediment), a preglomerular vasculitis should be considered.

Perhaps no tests are more helpful in differentiating the patient with ARF from one with pre- or postrenal azotemia than the simultaneous determination in the blood and urine of various chemical parameters (Table 3-4.) The value of such tests is based on the concept that renal tubular integrity is maintained in patients with prerenal azotemia whereas it is lost in those with ARF. Therefore, the ability to appropriately reabsorb salt, water, and urea should be clearly evident in patients with ECV depletion (i.e., prerenal azotemia).

Water reabsorption is measured by urinary specific gravity, or more accurately, by osmolarity. ECV depletion is a potent stimulus for water reabsorption, causing patients with prerenal azotemia to have a high urinary-specific gravity (>1.024) and osmolarity (400 ± 20 mOsm/L). Sodium reabsorption is likewise affected; the

Table 3-4 Diagnostic Indices in Acute Azotemia

	Prerenal Azotemia	ARF	Obstruction
S.G.	>1.024	1.015	1.015
U_{osm}	400 ± 20	300 ± 20	300 ± 40
U/P_{osm}	>1.5	1	1
U_{NA}	<20	>30	$<30^*$
FE_{NA}	$<1\%$	$>1\%$	$<1\%^*$
$U_{NA} \div U/P_{cr}$	<1	>1	<1
BUN:creatinine	20	10	$10-20^*$
U:P creatinine	>40	<20	<20

* First 24 hours.

urinary sodium concentration is usually less than 20 mEq/L with prerenal azotemia. Because tubular integrity is lost with ARF (particularly ARF caused by ATN), the urine can be neither concentrated nor diluted (specific gravity [SG] of 1.015 ± 0.004, osm. of 300 ± 20) and the ability to reabsorb sodium is lost ($U_{NA} > 30$ mEq/L)

Because urea is reabsorbed by the renal tubule but creatinine is not, conditions that increase tubular reabsorption, such as ECV contraction, will lead to a high blood urea: creatinine ratio (>20). Similarly, urinary creatinine is highly concentrated, with prerenal azotemia leading to a high urine:plasma creatinine ratio (>40). Patients with ARF will be unable to reabsorb urea selectively (BUN:creatinine ratio = 10) or concentrate urinary creatinine (urine:plasma creatinine ratio <20).

In an individual patient, however, the above-mentioned parameters often fail to distinguish ARF from prerenal azotemia. In patients with acute azotema, determining the fractional excretion of sodium (FE_{NA}) (the fraction of filtered sodium that is excreted) is very helpful. This measures the ratio of sodium excreted ($U_{NA} \cdot V$) to sodium filtered (plasma [Na] $\times$ GFR) by the following formula:

$$FE_{NA} = \cfrac{U_{NA} \cdot V}{P_{NA} \cdot \cfrac{(U_{cr} \cdot V)}{P_{cr}}}$$

where U = urine, P = plasma, V = volume.

Because the volumes cancel, the test can be done on a spot sample of urine and blood.

Individuals with a potent stimulus for sodium reabsorption (i.e., prerenal azotemia) should have a low level of sodium excretion and therefore a low FE_{NA} ($<1\%$). However, normal sodium reabsorption can be accomplished only with good tubular function. The patient with ARF will therefore be unable to increase sodium reabsorption and will demonstrate inappropriate sodium excretion ($FE_{NA} > 1\%$). When used properly, this test can differentiate ARF from prerenal azotemia in more than 90% of cases.

Several exceptions to the reliability of the FE_{NA} must be considered. Any condition decreasing sodium reabsorption (chronic renal insufficiency, diuretics, and glycosuria) will spuriously increase FE_{NA} and affect interpretation of the test, as well as that of most other urinary diagnostic tests. Conditions enhancing tubular sodium reabsorption (severe congestive failure, ascites, and nephrotic syndrome) will likewise spuriously lower the FE_{NA} in patients with ARF. In addition, acute glomerulonephritis, radiographic contrast agents, rhabdomyolysis, and occasionally sepsis are causes of ARF that are often associated with a low FE_{NA}. With these exceptions, the FE_{NA} can be effectively used to differentiate ARF and prerenal azotemia accurately.

Urinary tract obstruction is less well differentiated with the above indices. Early in the course of obstructive uropathy, particularly during the first 24 hours, urinary indices may mimic those of prerenal azotemia. However, they are soon indistinguishable from ARF. Therefore, the value of early radiographic visualization of the urinary tract to exclude obstruction in individuals with acute azotemia cannot be overemphasized.

Diagnostic Approach to Acute Azotemia

The diagnostic approach to acute azotemia is outlined in Figure 3-3 and Table 3-5. First, an artifactual cause of azotemia can be excluded by determining whether the patient has a history of using drugs known to influence serum creatinine spuriously (trimethoprim, cimetidine, cefoxitin) and whether the patient has factors spuriously increasing blood urea (use of corticosteroids, hyperalimentation, gastrointestinal bleeding). A serum assay for CPK can exclude creatinine overproduction from rhabdomyolysis.

Next, a search for urinary tract obstruction should exclude postrenal azotemia. For this, a Foley catheter and renal ultrasonography is adequate in most cases. An abdominal CT scan (without contrast material) can also be used to evaluate the retroperitoneum and reveal a cause for the obstruction, if found. In patients with only one kidney, a retrograde pyelogram may be necessary to exclude postrenal azotemia completely.

Prerenal azotemia is excluded by the physical examination, urine sediment, urine chemistries (particularly FE_{NA}), and occasionally

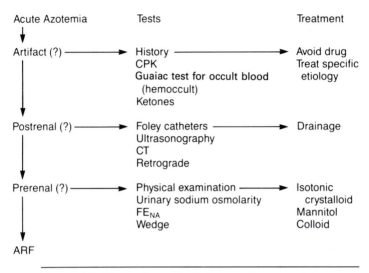

Figure 3-3: Diagnostic and basic therapeutic approach to patients with acute azotemia.

the pulmonary artery wedge pressure (PAWP). If prerenal azotemia is identified, patients should be treated aggressively with isotonic crystalloid solutions (normal saline or lactated Ringer's at 200 to 400 ml/hr) or mannitol (12.5 to 25 g IV bolus) until one sees a clinical response of increasing urine volume, physical findings of extracellular volume overload, or a PAWP of 18 to 20 mm Hg. If urine volume has not increased substantially, a large IV dose of furosemide (200 to 600 mg over 20 minutes) can be used in an attempt to "open up" the kidney and establish a diuresis. Low-dose dopamine infusion (2 to 3 μg/kg/min) may enhance renal perfusion and augment urine volume, as well. Even if the patient has established ARF at this point, the prognosis is improved when oliguria is avoided.

Only after one excludes artifactual, postrenal, and prerenal causes of acute azotemia can one consider the differential diagnostic approach to ARF (Fig. 3-4).

Table 3-5 Diagnostic Approach to Acute Azotemia

Consider artifact

Exclude obstruction:
    Foley catheter
    Ultrasonography
    CT (without contrast)
    Retrograde pyelogram

Exclude Prerenal azotemia
    Physical examination
    Diagnostic indices (Table 4-2)
    CVP or wedge pressure

Consider the cause of ARF (GN vs IN vs vascular)
    History
    UA
    Serologic studies
    Perfusion scan
    ?Biopsy

Consider ATN

Causes of Acute Renal Failure

The causes of ARF can be easily divided into four groups corresponding to the four major structures in the kidney. Abnormalities of the glomeruli (glomerulonephritis), interstitium (interstitial nephritis), blood vessels (vascular disease), or tubules (acute tubular necrosis [ATN]) are all possible causes of ARF. Of these, ATN accounts for the majority of ARF. Table 3-6 categorizes the common causes of ARF, several of which deserve particular mention.

Glomerular Hemodynamics

Aberrations of *glomerular hemodynamics* are an increasingly recognized cause of ARF. The GFR is dependent on four factors: (1) renal blood flow, (2) the hydrostatic pressures and (3) oncotic pressures in the glomerular capillary, and (4) the per-

ARF	Tests	Differential Diagnosis
Glomerular (?) →	History/physical examination → Sediment Cultures ANA, C_3, C_4 Biopsy (±)	Hemodynamic: Drugs, Hepatorenal; GN: SLE, Infectious, Rapidly progressive GN, Idiopathic
↓ Interstitial (?) →	History/physical examination → Eosinophilia Eosinophiluria Sediment Biopsy (±)	Allergic Pyelonephritis Crystals Myeloma
↓ Vascular (?) →	History/physical examination → Nuclear scan Arteriogram (±) Microangiopathic blood smear	Hypertension Thrombosis/embolus Cholesterol embolic Vasculitis Microangiopathy
↓ ATN →	History →	Ischemia: Shock, Sepsis; Toxic: Drugs, Contrast, Myoglobin

Figure 3-4: Diagnostic approach to patients with ARF (other causes of acute azotemia excluded). SLE = systemic lupus erythematosus. RPGN = rapidly progressive glomerulonephritis.

meability of the capillary membrane. Normally the GFR is the result of the homeostatic interaction of all these factors, with an increase in one often offsetting a decrease in another. In certain clinical situations, however, the GFR may become so critically dependent on a single factor that its interruption produces an abrupt and marked decrease in GFR (i.e., ARF). Thus, angiotensin converting enzyme (ACE) inhibitors can dilate the efferent capillary sphincter, decreasing glomerular hydrostatic pressure and GFR in patients with bilateral renal artery stenosis or severe congestive

Table 3-6 Etiology of Acute Renal Failure

Glomerular disease
  Hemodynamic changes
    Hepatorenal
    NSAIDs
    ACE inhibitors
    Nifedipine
    Nitroprusside
  Nephritic syndrome
    Bacterial endocarditis
    Systemic vasculitis
    Other infections
      Klebsiella abdominal abscess
      Hepatitis B
      "Shunt" nephritis
      Post-streptococcal
  Rapidly progressive (crescentic) GN
    Goodpasture's syndrome
    Nephritic diseases
    Vasculitis
    Idiopathic
      Immune complex
      Nonimmune deposits
      Antiglomerular basement membrane

Interstitial nephritis
  Drug-induced
    Antibiotics (penicillins, sulfonamides, cephalosporins)
    NSAIDs
    Diuretics
  Infections (pyelonephritis)
  Immune
    SLE
    Sjögren's syndrome
    Renal transplant rejection
  Infiltrative
    Leukemia, lymphoma
    Sarcoidosis
  Tubular obstruction
    Uric acid
    Oxalate (ethylene glycol)
    Myeloma kidney

Table 3-6 (Continued)

Vascular disease
  Renal artery disease
    Atherosclerotic
      Occlusion (thrombosis)
      Embolus
      Diffuse atherosclerotic (cholesterol) emboli
    Hypertensive
      Malignant hypertension
      Scleroderma crisis
    Traumatic (avulsion, intimal flap)
  Renal venous occlusion (thrombosis, ligation)
  TTP
  Vasculitis
    Polyarteritis
    Wegener's granulomatosis
    Henoch-Schönlein purpura
    Hypersensitivity vasculitis

ATN
  Ischemia
    Hemorrhage
    Hypotension/shock
    Sepsis
    Progressive prerenal azotemia (?)
    Obstetric complications
  Toxin-induced
    Drugs
      Antibiotics (aminoglycosides)
      Chemotherapy (*cis*-platinum, methotrexate, mitomycin)
      Anesthetics (methoxyflurane)
    Rhabdomyolysis/myoglobinuria
    Transfusion reaction
    Radiographic contrast agents
    Metals (Pb, Cd, arsenic, gold, Hg, platinum)
    Solvents (CCl$_4$, ethylene glycol, hydrocarbons)

SLE = systemic lupus erythematosus; TTP = thrombotic thrombocytopenic purpura; NSAIDS = Nonsteroidal anti-inflammatory drugs.

failure. In patients with cirrhosis or congestive failure, nonsteroidal anti-inflammatory drugs (NSAIDs) can cause ARF by compromising renal blood flow. Severe afferent arteriolar vasoconstriction believed to occur with the hepatorenal syndrome can produce ARF by decreasing renal blood flow and glomerular hydrostatic pressure. Even sudden increases in plasma oncotic pressure or decrements in glomerular capillary permeability (caused by hypercalcemia, aminoglycosides, aspirin) may cause ARF in certain patients. Finally, a few reports have implicated potent vasodilators such as nifedipine and nitroprusside as a cause of ARF.

The ARF caused by these changes in glomerular hemodynamics is usually functional. When drug-induced, it is often dose-related and can be reversed soon after the cause is eliminated. Renal biopsy shows normal histology.

Acute Glomerulonephritis

Acute glomerulonephritis may also cause ARF. Patients with acute glomerulonephritis will usually have either nephritic syndrome or rapidly progressive glomerulonephritis (see Chapter 4). The presence of hematuria (particularly if dysmorphic RBCs or RBC casts are seen), albuminuria, and hypertension should alert the clinician to this possibility. ANA and complement levels can usually exclude lupus. Blood cultures are necessary to evaluate an infectious cause. One must also search for historical or physical clues to a systemic vasculitis or Goodpasture's syndrome. When the exact etiology of ARF cannot be readily established and/or the patient shows signs of glomerulonephritis (GN), an early renal biopsy should be considered.

Interstitial Nephritis

Interstitial nephritis is another cause of ARF. Most cases of interstitial nephritis are drug-related, caused by antibiotics (penicillins, sulfonamides, and cephalosporins) or the nonsteroidal anti-inflammatory drugs. Fever, rash, eosinophilia, and eosinophiluria often accompany ARF. Acute pyelonephritis may occasionally cause ARF, although this is not the typical clinical course. In addition, crystal-induced (uric acid, oxalate) interstitial nephritis or myeloma kidney may be encountered in a patient with ARF. In these cases, often the clinician must rely on a high index of suspicion and careful urinalysis (demonstrating pyuria, WBC casts, and eosinophils) in order to confirm the diagnosis.

Vascular Diseases

Vascular disease of the kidney is a less common cause of ARF. Nevertheless, when it does occur, it is usually an extremely serious condition and therefore should be diligently sought and excluded. In the elderly population, arteriosclerotic disease of the large vessels causing renal artery occlusion or embolus may be most likely. The latter is certainly more common in individuals with recurrent cardiac arrhythmias. Diffuse embolization of cholesterol plaque from damaged arteries after a major vascular procedure can also cause ARF and is often difficult to distinguish from systemic vasculitis. Trauma may also be a serious cause of renal vascular insult. This mandates a complete evaluation of any patient with major or minor trauma showing hematuria in the urinary sediment. Systemic vasculitis may present with ARF. These syndromes are usually readily apparent by their systemic nature, active urinary sediment, and other specific nonrenal manifestations, depending on the individual syndrome. Finally, diseases of the microcirculation should be considered in any patient with ARF, thrombopenia, hemolysis, or accelerated hypertension (see Chapter 6).

Acute Tubular Necrosis

ATN accounts for nearly 80% of all ARF. ATN is usually caused by either an ischemic or a toxic insult. In general, ischemic causes are more serious, with a higher incidence of oliguria and a more prolonged clinical course. Severe hemorrhage, hypotension, shock, and septicemia are typical examples of ischemic insults.

Table 3-7 Factors Affecting the Nephrotoxicity of Aminoglycosides

Dose: direct relationship

Duration: direct relationship

Dosing interval: constant infusion>t.i.d.>b.i.d.>daily

Individual drug: gentamicin>tobramycin>amikacin>netilmicin

Prolonged and significant prerenal azotemia can also probably lead to ATN. Obstetrical catastrophes appear to be one cause of ischemic acute renal failure that has an excellent clinical outcome, probably owing to the patient's youth and general good health.

The common toxins causing ATN are listed in Table 3-6. Of these, aminoglycoside antibiotics and iodinated radiographic contrast agents remain the most common.

The nephrotoxic potential of aminoglycosides is related to several factors, including the individual agent, the dose, the dosing frequency, and the duration of therapy (Table 3-7). Several studies, however, dissociate nephrotoxicity to the aminoglycoside serum level (making suspect the practice of monitoring drug levels to avoid nephrotoxicity). In addition, several factors may predispose a patient to aminoglycoside toxicity, including advanced age, pre-existing renal disease, intravascular volume contraction, hypokalemia, and the concomitant use of other nephrotoxins. Recognition of these factors is extremely important as it may enable the physician to prevent ATN.

Iodinated radiographic contrast agents are a common nephrotoxin, particularly in diabetics, whose nephrotoxic potential is directly related to the patient's baseline serum creatinine. The elderly, individuals with multiple myeloma or intravascular volume depletion, may also be at great risk for dye-induced ATN. Iodinated radiographic contrast agents are among the few toxic causes of ATN associated with a low fractional excretion of sodium (FE_{NA}).

NSAIDs do not usually cause ATN. The nephrologic syndromes associated with NSAIDs include the following:

1. Salt and water retention.
2. Functional decrease in GFR.

3. Nephrotic syndrome.
4. Acute interstitial nephritis.
5. Hyporeninemic hypoaldosteronism.

Most commonly, salt and water retention occurs, causing clinical edema and exacerbating hypertension. A reduction in nonsteroidal drugs and/or an increase in antihypertensives is often necessary. As mentioned, functional decrements in GFR are often noted when nonsteroidal drugs are given to patients whose renal blood flow is critically dependent on prostaglandins (those who have congestive failure, cirrhosis, ECV depletion). The nephrotic syndrome (usually minimal-change disease) can be seen to occur with the use of several agents in this group often associated simultaneously with acute interstitial nephritis. Finally, nonsteroidal drugs inhibit renin release (by inhibiting prostaglandins), which may cause severe hyperkalemia.

Despite years of clinical and laboratory research, the pathophysiologic mechanisms responsible for ARF remain unclear. Most investigators, however, believe that the factors responsible for the initiation of ARF are not necessarily those involved in its maintenance. Initially, cellular damage is believed to arise from either an ischemic or toxic insult, altering cellular transport functions and causing eventual necrosis. (The exact mechanism may differ depending on the etiology of ARF.) In most experimental models, the result has been a decrease in renal blood flow and glomerular filtration. The mechanism by which tubular damage causes a decrement of GFR is unknown.

Although the initiating factors may resolve within 24 hours, the clinical course of oliguric ARF is maintained for a prolonged period (usually 12 to 21 days). Several theories have been proposed to explain this "maintenance" phase of ARF (Table 3-8). Although support can be found for all factors demonstrated in a variety of experimental settings, the exact mechanism or mechanisms responsible for the maintenance of ARF in most cases remain unknown.

Of perhaps more interest is the mechanism responsible for the nonoliguria in some patients with ARF. Urinary volume is the sum of the volume filtered minus the volume reabsorbed by the tubules. Thus, nonoliguria could result from either of two situations: relative

Table 3-8 Factors Responsible for Maintenance of ARF

Tubular factors
  Back-leak of ultrafiltrate
  Tubular obstruction

Hemodynamic factors
  Afferent arteriolar vasoconstriction
    Renin-angiotensin vasoconstriction
    Swollen endothelial cells
    Lack of vasodilator (prostaglandin [?], kinin [?])
    ADH
  Efferent arteriolar vasodilation

Glomerular factors
  Decreased permeability
  Decreased surface area

preservation of tubular reabsorption with less severe reduction in GFR or reduction in both tubular reabsorption and GFR. Experimental evidence suggests that nonoliguria results from the former. Indeed, when compared with oliguric patients, nonoliguric patients have higher GFRs and a lower FE_{NA} (i.e., greater tubular reabsorption). Whether this is the result of a less severe insult or a different pathophysiology is unknown.

From the clinical standpoint, patients with nonoliguric ARF certainly have a more benign lesion. Compared with oliguric patients, patients with nonoliguria have fewer morbid complications (gastrointestinal bleeding, sepsis, neurologic abnormalities), shorter hospital stays, a reduced dialysis requirement, and most importantly, an improved survival rate.

Diagnostic Approach to Acute Renal Failure

Once ARF has been established, the clinician should consider the least likely diagnoses first. Together, GN, interstitial nephritis, and vascular diseases account for fewer than 30% of cases of ARF. They can be distinguished by a careful history, physical examination, and urinalysis. GN should be considered first. A urine sediment showing dysmorphic RBCs or RBC casts makes this diagnosis likely. A serologic search will usually exclude lupus. Hypocomplementemia, the history, and physical examination will evaluate bacterial endocarditis, occult visceral abscess, or "shunt nephritis." If doubt remains as to the etiology of GN, a renal biopsy may be helpful.

Next, one should consider acute interstitial nephritis. Fever, rash, eosinophilia, and eosinophiluria suggests a drug reaction, most commonly due to antibiotics, nonsteroidal drugs, or diuretics (although eosinophilia and eosinophiluria are less commonly seen with nonsteroidal drugs). The history, physical examination, and urine sediment (pyuria, bacteriuria, WBC casts) can exclude pyelonephritis. Uric acid or oxalate crystals are important diagnostic clues as well. Multiple myeloma, which may present initially as ARF, should also be considered.

Primary vascular diseases are the easiest causes of ARF to overlook. Once they are considered, however, renal thromboembolism, cholesterol embolism, or vasculitis are not difficult diagnoses to make. Thromboembolism causes flank pain, fever, hypertension, hematuria, and a rise in serum lactate dehydrogenase (LDH). The cholesterol emboli syndrome may mimic systemic vasculitis, but a history of recent intra-arterial procedure or anticoagulation will be helpful. The systemic vasculitides affecting the kidney can be differentiated based on their clinical and laboratory features (see Chapter 6, Table 6-6).

Finally, one should consider the various ischemic and toxic causes of ATN. These are largely distinguished by the patient's history.

Prevention of Acute Renal Failure

ARF can often be prevented by identifying and avoiding certain key risk factors. Table 3-9 lists several of these potential risk factors and gives suggestions for minimizing their adverse effects on the kidney. Clearly, the most significant risk is decreased renal perfusion caused by absolute volume depletion (hemorrhage, gastrointestinal losses) or "third space" fluids in patients who have

Table 3-9 Potential Risk Factors for the Development of ARF and Suggestions for Their Minimization

Risk Factor	Suggestions to Minimize Risk
Decreased renal perfusion	
Absolute ECV depletion	Isotonic crystalloids
Cardiac failure	Inotropic agents; low-dose dopamine
"Third space"	Colloids; isotonic crystalloids
Cirrhosis, ascites	Low-dose dopamine
Positive pressure ventilation	Limit if possible; expand ECV
Previous/concurrent nephrotoxins	Use of alternative agent if possible
Aminoglycosides	Expand dosing interval; adjust dose
Radiocontrast	Expand ECV/mannitol; limit dye volume
NSAIDs	Avoid use
Chemotherapy	Expand ECV
Pre-existing renal insufficiency	Expand ECV if possible; adjust dose of potential nephrotoxins
Electrolyte abnormalities	
Hypokalemia	Correct
Hypophosphatemia	Correct
Hypercalcemia	Saline diuresis; avoid use of phosphorus
Hyperalimentation (?)	Limit protein as much as possible (?)
Increased abdominal pressure (?)	Decompress (?)

undergone surgery or have multiple trauma. ECV expansion with isotonic crystalloid solutions and/or colloids can greatly minimize this risk. Low-dose dopamine infusions (1.5 to 3 μg/kg/min) may abrogate the decrement in renal blood flow seen in patients with cardiac failure or cirrhosis with ascites. Lastly, positive end-expiratory pressure (PEEP) and other forms of positive pressure ventilation may compromise cardiac output and renal perfusion. If possible, one should minimize PEEP and expand the ECV with crystalloids in high-risk patients.

If a patient has recently received a potential nephrotoxin, an alternative agent should be selected if possible. Fortunately, several excellent antibiotics are available that provide comparable antimicrobial coverage to the aminoglycosides. If one must use an aminoglycoside in a high-risk patient, expanding the dosing interval (to roughly eight times the serum creatinine) and closely following urinary volumes and serum creatinines is of value. Polyuria or an increased serum creatinine should prompt a further widening of the dosing interval or discontinuation of the drug. Although a "peak" aminoglycoside level will serve to guide therapy, there is little evidence that a "trough" level will allow one to minimize or avoid nephrotoxicity. The routine use of aminoglycoside levels as guides to therapy is therefore unnecessary.

There is substantial literature suggesting that radiographic contrast nephrotoxicity can be minimized in some patients by avoiding volume depletion and administering mannitol and crystalloids after the dye study. Recent studies have also documented that atrial natriuretic peptide (a potent renal vasodilator) is also protective at this time. Limiting dye volume to less than 125 ml and avoiding multiple contrast studies within 24 to 36 hours will also minimize the risk. There is no evidence that nonionic or low molecular weight IV contrast agents reduce their nephrotoxic potential.

Recent studies suggest that hyperalimentation poses a risk for ARF. In one study, rats fed a high-protein diet had a significantly higher mortality than those fed a low- or zero-protein diet after a comparable renal ischemic insult. Perhaps minimizing protein intake to 0.6 to 0.8 g/kg/day or less in certain high-risk patients would be beneficial.

Although some data exist supporting abdominal decompression as a means of improving renal perfusion in patients with ileus or tense ascites, the clinician must be very cautious about massive paracenteses (0.5 to 1 L or greater). Ascitic fluid may rapidly reaccumulate at the expense of the intravascular volume, precipitating abrupt renal shutdown.

In more than 60% of ARF cases, more than one risk factor is identified. This is particularly true in certain patients, such as those undergoing aortic aneurysectomy or cardiopulmonary bypass, those with prolonged respiratory failure, and those who have had multiple trauma or severe burns. In these patients, the clinician must be particularly cautious of potential nephrotoxins and diligent in correcting the other potential renal risk factors outlined in Table 3-9.

Treatment and Prognosis of Acute Renal Failure

As outlined in the previous section, prevention of ARF is the best form of therapy. Nevertheless, once ARF is established, several treatment modalities are important. These can be divided into four categories, including conversion of oliguria to nonoliguria, prevention of complications, supportive or expectant management, and specific therapy for ARF per se (see Table 3-10).

Table 3-10 General Treatment Principles of ARF

Convert to "oliguria"
  Correct ECV deficits
  Furosemide (200 to 400 mg slow IV)
  Dopamine (1.5 to 3.0 μg/kg/min)

Prevent common complications
  Sepsis
    Limit number/duration of lines
    Use antibiotics prudently
    Minimize use of immunosuppressives
    Perform periodic "blind" cultures?
    Limit nasotracheal intubation?
  Gastrointestinal ulceration
    Gastric suction/antacids
    H_2 blockers
    Sucralfate
  Drug adjustments
    Meperidine
    Diazepam
    Procainamide/NAPA
    Metabolic loads
      Na (sodium polystyrene sulfonate [Kayexalate], carbenicillin, ticarcillin)
      K (penicillin K)
      Mg (antacids)
Provide supportive care
  Dialysis (hemodialysis versus peritoneal dialysis versus CAVH)
  Hyperalimentation
Initiate specific therapy
  ANF?
  Prostaglandin analogs?
  Oxygen scavengers?

Oliguria Versus Nonoliguria

Compared with oliguric patients, nonoliguric patients have significantly fewer complications (gastrointestinal bleeding, sepsis, acidosis), briefer hospital stays, and an improved survival rate. In most clinical series, the mortality rate of patients with nonoliguric ARF is half that of oliguric patients. This improvement appears to reflect more than simply a less severe form of ARF (resulting from a less severe insult) in the nonoliguric patients. Rather, the diuresis simplifies management, lessens the requirement for dialysis (avoiding additional invasive procedures and heparinization), and allows for improved nutritional support. Therefore, whenever possible, the clinician should attempt to induce a diuresis and "convert" those patients with oliguria to nonoliguria. In order to accomplish this, one must first be sure that volume deficits are corrected. Renal vasodilatory doses of dopamine (1.5 to 3 μg/kg/min) may be tried. Finally, high-dose loop diuretics (furosemide, 200 to 400 mg IV over 20 minutes) may prompt a substantial diuresis in some oliguric patients.

Common Complications

Preventing the *common complications* of ARF may do more to improve survival than any specific treatment. Chief among these complications is sepsis. Limiting the number and duration of central venous and arterial catheters will greatly minimize this risk. So, too, will the prudent use of corticosteroids, other immunosuppressives, and broad-spectrum antibiotics, all of which enhance the likelihood of the development of resistant bacteria and fungal organisms; at least one study has directly correlated mortality in ARF with the number of antibiotics administered. Periodic "blind" cultures of blood, sputum, and urine may be helpful with early identification of occult sepsis. Prolonged nasotracheal intubation can predispose to serious sinusitis and subsequent septicemia.

Prophylaxis for gastric stress ulceration is extremely important. Frequent antacids (which keep gastric pH >4.5), H_2 receptor blockers, and sucralfate all appear to be effective measures. A slightly greater incidence of nosocomial pneumonias in patients given H_2 receptor blockers may reflect bacterial growth in the stomach as gastric pH rises. Although preliminary, these data suggest fewer complications when sucralfate is used for ulcer prophylaxis.

Dosage adjustment for several commonly prescribed drugs is necessary. Excellent reviews are published on this subject, but a few drugs require special comments. Meperidine hydrochloride should be avoided in patients with renal failure since its metabolite (normeperidine) accumulates, causing seizures. Metabolites of valium may cause profound sedation for days to weeks in patients with ARF. N-acetylated procainamide (NAPA) may accumulate in patients with renal failure who are receiving procainamide and produce polymorphic ventricular tachycardia. Because of decreased protein-binding in uremic patients, the pharmacologic effect is greater than usual for any given dose of morphine, necessitating dosage adjustment in ARF. Finally, one must often avoid the hidden metabolic loads of sodium (sodium polystyrene sulfonate [Kayexalate], carbenicillin, ticarcillin), potassium (penicillin K), and magnesium (antacids) which may be administered.

Supportive Care

Supportive care centers around fluid management, dialysis, and nutritional support. Hemodialysis or peritoneal dialysis is indicated whenever uremic complications develop (e.g., myoclonus, seizures, lethargy, pericarditis) or when fluid overload, acidosis, and hyperkalemia are refractory to medical management. Once initiated, dialysis should be performed frequently enough to control these symptoms and keep the BUN under 100 mg/dl. There is no evidence to support that "early" or "aggressive" dialysis (keeping the urea at less than 30 mg/dl) offers any advantage over the conventional approach. For patients whose major problem is excess ECV, particularly those with severe cardiac failure, continuous arteriovenous hemofiltration (CAVH) offers some advantage.

Hyperalimentation has been shown to have a favorable influence on the prognosis of ARF in both clinical and animal studies. Whenever possible, this should be accomplished enterally. Three basic requirements will guide the specific formula in a given patient: (1) protein intake must be 0.8 to 1.5 g/kg/day, (2) nonprotein calories must be at least 140 calories/g (N = protein ÷ 6.25), and (3) lipid content must not exceed 40% of total calories. One should avoid standard parenteral solutions and selectively add electrolytes, calcium, phosphorus, magnesium, vitamins, and insulin as needed. Essential amino acid solutions (Nephramine, Aminosyn-RF) are not routinely needed, although an occasional patient may benefit from them (usually when trying to avoid dialysis).

Specific Therapy

Although some patients with GN, interstitial nephritis, and vascular disease may respond to a specific therapy, little is available for patients with ATN. However, several recent studies show amelioration of ATN with renal vasodilators such as atrial natriuretic factor (ANF) and the oral prostaglandin E analog misoprostol. In addition, oxygen-free radical scavengers may improve renal recovery after an ischemic insult. Thus, the future holds promise for a more specific treatment of ATN.

Despite the preventative and therapeutic measures outlined above, the mortality rate of ARF remains 50% overall, 60 to 70% in oliguric patients, and greater than 70% in those with multiple organ failure. In survivors, however, the chances for renal recovery are excellent (greater than 90%). Like the patient survival rate, the ultimate renal survival rate is dependent on the cause of ARF with prolonged ischemic insults yielding the worst prognosis. In 80% of patients, the time to renal recovery is less than 30 days. Virtually all of those recovering function will do so within 8 weeks.

Case 3-1: *Discussion*

1. This is certainly acute azotemia. After an artifact has been excluded, one should consider prerenal azotemia, postrenal azotemia, and ARF as possible diagnoses.

2. Although unlikely in this case, bladder outlet obstruction should be excluded by a Foley catheter and imaging of the urinary tract, usually ultrasonography.

3. Prerenal azotemia can be distinguished from ARF by several diagnostic and physical indices. In this patient the BUN to serum creatinine ratio was 24, the urine sodium was 2 mEq/L, the urine osmolarity was 550 mOsm/L and the FE_{NA} was 0.03%. Prerenal azotemia is therefore the most likely cause of his acute azotemia. The prerenal azotemia could be caused by the low intravascular volume or poor cardiac output. In this case, the 5-kg decline in weight implies that it is the former. In certain cases, however, determination of pulmonary artery wedge pressure will be needed to differentiate between these two possibilities. Hypokalemia and metabolic alkalosis suggest overdiuresis in this patient. The hyponatremia is likely related to furosemide-induced renal salt loss as well as to nonosmotic ADH secretion and a degree in delivery of filtrate to the diluting nephron segment (see Chapter 8).

Case 3-2: *Discussion*

1. Despite severe azotemia, the well-preserved hemoglobin and hematocrit suggest acute azotemia. Previous laboratory values should be sought and renal size determined to confirm the acute process.

2. Possible diagnoses include artifact, prerenal azotemia, postrenal azotemia, and ARF. Because of its reversibility, obstructive uropathy must always be considered early and excluded.

3. Foley catheterization should be performed. In this patient, it resulted in a brisk diuresis and resolution of azotemia (to creatinine of 1.9 mg/dl). If no improvement in output or azotemia had occurred after catheter insertion, it would have needed to be removed. If the patient had not been obstructed, urinary diagnostic indices and exclusion of prerenal azotemia would have been the next diagnostic step.

Case 3-3: *Discussion*

1. This patient developed worsening renal insufficiency during hospitalization. This is usually related to volume factors (prerenal azotemia) or a toxin (ARF). The excellent urine volume

(1500 ml/day) tends to exclude the former and suggests nonoliguric ARF. ARF may be caused by glomerular, interstitial, vascular, or tubular damage. A diligent review of the urinary sediment should exclude GN and vasculitis (by demonstrating absence of casts or hematuria) and interstitial nephritis (by demonstrating absence of pyuria or WBC casts). Renal perfusion radioisotope renogram should be obtained to exclude severe vascular compromise. Therefore in this patient, ATN is the likely cause. The most probable cause of this ATN is an iodinated radiographic contrast agent. Diabetics are at high risk for this complication.

2. This "contrast nephropathy" can be avoided or abrogated by maintaining intravascular volume, avoiding dehydration, and perhaps administering mannitol soon after the contrast is given.

3. Only supportive fluid therapy was given. "Contrast nephropathy" will usually resolve within 3 to 7 days without specific therapy.

4. This patient most likely has underlying diabetic nephropathy. Documentation of nephrotic range proteinuria, proliferative retinopathy, normal renal size, and otherwise bland urinary sediment would confirm this suspicion without renal biopsy.

5. In diabetics, hyperkalemic hyperchloremic non-anion gap acidosis is usually caused by hyporeninemic hypoaldosteronism.

Case 3-4: *Discussion*
1. This patient likely had acute azotemia on admission which worsened despite correction of his acute abdominal process. Although he was receiving cefoxitin postoperatively, which can artifactually raise serum creatinine, the rise in both urea and creatinine as well as oliguria suggests a more significant process. Obstruction should be ruled out with an ultrasound examination.

Although the patient's weight increased postoperatively, prerenal azotemia must still be strongly considered. This and ARF are the most likely causes for the azotemia.

2. In acutely oliguric, azotemic patients, urine chemistries are invaluable. In this patient, the urine sodium was 4 mEq/L, the specific gravity was 1.032, osmolarity was 495 mOsm/L, and the calculated FE_{NA} was 0.02%. These values strongly suggest prerenal azotemia, probably caused by "third space" volume and decreased intravascular volume. An isotonic fluid challenge and/or administration of mannitol is therefore warranted.

However, the above urine chemistries are not atypical for acute GN. In addition, one must not forget that an intra-abdominal abscess can cause acute GN. If the patient does not adequately respond to fluid administration or if the urinalysis shows RBC casts, this diagnosis should be strongly considered.

3. The metabolic acidosis is of the high anion gap variety suggesting lactate, ketones, or a toxin such as salicylate, methanol, ethylene glycol, or paraldehyde. This degree of azotemia is not enough to account for a uremic acidosis.

Case 3-5: *Discussion*

The patient was not receiving any medications to affect his BUN or creatinine level artifactually. On the first day of hospitalization, an ultrasound examination showed two normal-sized kidneys without obstruction. Prerenal azotemia can be excluded by the physical examination, as well as by the fact that the patient had a good urine output and FE_{NA} of 1.1%.

This patient therefore appears to have established ARF. The history and urinalysis fail to point to a specific cause. Serum and urine protein electrophoresis and immunoelectrophoresis failed to show a paraprotein. However, serologic studies revealed a C3 55 mg/dl (normal range is 84 to 210 mg/dl), C4 20 mg/dl (normal range is 12 to 50 mg/dl), ANA 1:2560 and anti-DNA 1:20 (normal is 0 to 10). Cryoglobulins were negative. No obvious cause for toxic or ischemic ATN was identified.

A renal biopsy revealed crescentic (4/9) GN without vasculitis. Lymphoma cell infiltrates could not be identified. Immunologic staining was positive for complement and IgG in a focal mesangial distribution.

The patient's renal function failed to improve, despite therapy with high-dose steroids, alkylating agents, plasmapheresis, and primary treatment for lymphoma.

Rapidly progressive, crescentic GN has rarely been reported with lymphoma. Presumably this process is related to a lymphoma cell antigen. The patient did not appear to have clinical lupus, although the high ANA titer and positive anti-DNA are certainly suggestive of that disease.

Case 3-6: *Discussion*

1. Diagnostic steps should include abdominal ultrasonography, cystoscopy with retrograde pyelography attempt and transperineal needle biopsy of the prostate. In this patient, abdominal ultrasonography revealed slightly enlarged kidneys with pyelocaliectasis and ureterectasis down to the level of the pelvic brim. Cystoscopy revealed elevation of the bladder neck and trigone by a mass that invaded the bladder and made identification of the ureteral orifices impossible. Transperineal needle biopsy of the prostate revealed adenocarcinoma of the prostate on frozen-section microscopic examination, and bilateral orchiectomies were performed. A percutaneous nephrostomy tube was placed in the right kidney and a diuresis was ensured. Five days later, the patient began passing urine through his bladder, a percutaneous nephrostogram revealed resolution of the ureteral obstruction, and the tube was removed.

2. This patient had acute postrenal failure because of adenocarcinoma of the prostate that was hormone-sensitive. The anemia was caused by bone marrow involvement.

References

Anderson RJ, Linas SL, Berns AS, et al. Nonoliguric acute renal failure. N Engl J Med 1977; 296:1134–1138.

Dixon BS, Anderson RJ. Nonoliguric acute renal failure. Am J Kidney Dis 1985; 6:71–80.

Espinel CH, Gregory AA. Differential diagnosis of acute renal failure. Clin Neph 1980; 13:73.

Henrich WL. Nephrotoxicity of nonsteroidal anti-inflammatory agents. Am J Kidney Dis 1983; 2:478–484.

Hou SH, Burshinsky DA, Wish JB. Hospital acquired renal insufficiency: a prospective study. Am J Med 1983; 74:243.

Miller PD, Krebs RA, Neal BJ, et al. Polyuric prerenal failure. Arch Int Med 1980; 140:907–909.

Myers BD, Hilberman M, Carrie BJ, et al. Dynamics of glomerular ultrafiltration following open-heart surgery. Kidney Int 1981; 20: 366–374.

Rasmussen HH, Ibels LS. Acute renal failure: multivariate analysis of causes and risk factors. Am J Med 1982; 73:211.

4 Glomerulonephritis

- Case Presentations

- Classifications of Glomerulonephritis

- Nephrotic Syndrome

- Nephritic Syndrome

- Rapidly Progressive Glomerulonephritis

- Chronic Glomerulonephritis

- Diagnostic Approach

- Case Discussions

Case 4-1

A 57-year-old man presented with increasing edema. Urinalysis revealed 4 + protein (later quantitated at 5.5 g/24 hr) but was otherwise normal. Serum creatinine was 2.8 mg/dl; C_{cr} was 34 ml/minute; serum albumin was 3.0 mg/dl.

Twenty years earlier he had undergone a left nephrectomy because of chronic pain and a congenital ureteropelvic junction obstruction. Ten years earlier he had been refused insurance because of albuminuria. Five years earlier he had been told of glucose intolerance. For the past 3 years, he had been taking glyburide. He was not taking any other medications.

Physical examination showed the patient to be 5′10″ in height, with a weight of 98 kg and a blood pressure of 142/88. Fundi were grossly normal. No bruits were evident in the neck, abdomen, or legs, and 3+ peripheral and 1+ sacral edema was noted. A large right thyroid nodule was palpated.

Questions

1. What is the differential diagnosis?
2. Should a renal biopsy be performed?
3. What is the appropriate therapy?

Case 4-2

A previously well, 43-year-old woman suffered a flu-like illness 6 weeks earlier, characterized by sore throat, nausea, vomiting, and extreme fatigue. Coincident with resolution of her symptoms, she noted progressive edema. Two weeks earlier, she saw her doctor, who prescribed a diuretic antihypertensive agent (Maxide). BUN and creatinine at that time were 27 mg/dl and 1.1 mg/dl, respectively, and urine showed 4+ proteinuria.

Past history revealed obesity and degenerative arthritis, for which she had taken 600 mg of fenoprofen three times daily for 8 months.

Because of progressive edema and dyspnea, she was admitted to the hospital. She was afebrile, with a blood pressure of 164/98 and normal fundi. Her chest was clear except for bibasilar dullness, and there was 4+ peripheral and sacral edema. BUN and creatinine was 85 and 6.6, respectively. Urine protein was 12 g/24 hr. The urine sediment showed only a few granular casts without cells.

Questions

1. What is the cause of the nephrotic syndrome?
2. What is the cause of the ARF?
3. What treatment should be implemented?

Case 4-3

An 83-year-old woman was admitted for nausea and vomiting. She had been taking digoxin, potassium chloride, furosemide, and warfarin for compensated congestive heart failure. At 80 years of age, she had bacterial endocarditis necessitating aortic valve replacement. Three months earlier she uneventfully underwent cataract extraction. Her BUN was 12 mg/dl and her creatinine was 0.8 mg/dl at that time.

Physical examination revealed a blood pressure of 144/92, a temperature of 99°F and a regular pulse rate of 94 beats per minute. Chest examination showed bilateral basilar rales. The jugular venous pulse was 8 to 10 cm H_2O. Cardiac examination showed a 3/6 systolic ejection type murmur; there was no diastolic murmur. The skin was without lesions. Bruits were absent in the abdomen.

Laboratory tests revealed a sodium level of 143 mEq/L, a potassium level of 7.2 mEq/L, Cl level of 106 mEq/L, a bicarbonate radical (HCO_3) of 19 mEq/L, a BUN of 98 mg/dl, creatinine of 7.4 mg/dl, a digoxin level of 7, a WBC count of 9,300, a hemoglobin level of 10.4, a prothrombin (PT) of 11/16 and a partial thromboplastin time (PTT) of 68 seconds. The urinalysis showed 4+ proteinuria, 10 to 12 WBC/hpf, too numerous to count RBC/hpf, and numerous granular and RBC casts.

Three days after admission, the patient underwent a grand mal seizure. A CT scan of the brain was negative.

Questions

1. What is the glomerular syndrome?
2. What is the differential diagnosis?
3. What would you suspect on renal biopsy?

Few areas in nephrology generate more confusion than glomerulonephritis. The fact that glomerular diseases are variably classified according to their immunologic, histologic, or clinical features adds to this confusion. This chapter presents the varied classifications of the glomerulopathies, but focuses only on a *clinical classification* based on the clinical features that are seen at the time of presentation.

Classifications of Glomerulonephritis

Immune Classification

Table 4-1 classifies glomerular disease on the basis of the responsible immunologic mechanism. Glomerular diseases can be classified as immune complex disease, antiglomerular basement membrane (AGBM) disease, or cell-mediated disease. The major drawback of this approach is that many glomerulopathies (diabetes, amyloidosis, drug-induced) are not immune-mediated. Nevertheless, this approach offers the hope that particular (etiologic) antigens can eventually be identified and that specific treatment directed against these antigens can be developed. It therefore appears to be the classification of the future.

Most immune-mediated glomerular diseases involve immune complex formation. These complexes are identified by immunofluorescence microscopy as granular-appearing deposits in the mesangium and/or along the glomerular basement membrane. Traditionally, this was believed to involve the formation of antigen-antibody complexes in the serum (circulating immune complexes)

Table 4-1 Immunologic Classification of Glomerulonephritis

Immune complex disease
  Circulating immune complexes
    Berger's (IgA) nephritis
    Henoch-Schönlein purpura
    SLE nephritis
    Bacterial endocarditis
  In situ complex formation
    Post-streptococcal
    Membranous (?)

AGBM disease
  Goodpasture's syndrome
  Idiopathic RPGN

Cell-Mediated (?)
  Minimal-change disease (?)
  FSG (?)

SLE = systemic lupus erythematosus.

which deposited nonspecifically in the glomerulus. Now, however, it appears that a more frequent mechanism involves antibody-binding to a specific glomerular antigen (in situ complex formation). The antigen may be foreign, as in post-streptococcal GN, or native to the glomerulus and altered in some way. With both types of immune complexes, binding complement with subsequent activation of the complement cascade mediates the inflammatory process.

AGBM disease is easily identified by immunofluorescence microscopy by a smooth "ribbonlike" linear staining of immunoglobulin along the glomerular basement membrane (GBM). This is certainly the immune mechanism responsible for Goodpasture's syndrome, but is likely involved in other glomerulopathies, as well. Linear staining can also be seen in patients with diabetic nodular glomerulosclerosis (Kimmelstiel-Wilson disease), but is believed to be nonspecific only and not pathogenic in patients with this condition.

Although direct evidence is lacking, some glomerular diseases (minimal change GN and some forms of focal glomerulosclerosis) may be related to cell-mediated immunity. This may explain the not uncommon occurrence of minimal change GN with Hodgkin's disease. It also might explain why the proteinuria of lupus nephritis often improves after total lymphoid irradiation, despite the fact that there has been no change in histology.

Histologic Classification

The traditional approach to classifying glomerular diseases has been based on glomerular histology (usually by light microscopy). Terms like minimal change, focal sclerosis, proliferative and crescentic therefore become "diseases." Although very nonspecific and offering little hope of identifying the etiology, this classification system is extremely useful, particularly in classifying idiopathic or primary forms of GN. It allows the clinician to predict outcome and guide therapies, depending on the histologic category into which the patient falls. The major drawback to this approach, however, is that not all patients with GN undergo renal biopsy. Indeed, some clinicians have argued against the routine use of renal biopsy in favor of empiric therapeutic trials, even for adult patients with GN. Nevertheless, because diagnostic accuracy is low when the diagnosis is based on clinical features alone and because corticosteroids and cytotoxic agents have significant potential for serious side effects, we favor renal biospy in most patients with clinical signs of GN. The renal biopsy allows one to (1) make a specific diagnosis, (2) prognosticate better, and (3) guide immunosuppressive therapy.

Table 4-2 outlines the clinical characteristics of the idiopathic (primary) glomerulopathies according to the histologic classification. Each will be explored in more detail in subsequent sections of this chapter.

Clinical Classification

Based on their clinical features at presentation, patients with GN can be classified into five major syndromes (Table 4-3). These include (1) asymptomatic glomerular abnormalities, (2) nephrotic syndrome, (3) nephritic syndrome, (4) rapidly progressive GN (RPGN), and (5) chronic GN. The approach to patients with asymptomatic hematuria and/or proteinuria is outlined in Chapter 2. The other major syndromes as well as their common primary (idiopathic) and secondary (systemic) causes are outlined below.

Nephrotic Syndrome

The nephrotic syndrome is the clinical tetrad of major proteinuria (>3 to 3.5 g/day and/or urinary protein:creatinine index>3) and its consequent hypoalbuminemia, edema, and hyperlipidemia. The syndrome results from a major alteration in glomerular permeability due to structural damage of the glomerular capillary wall or loss of its negative charges. It may be caused by a variety of primary renal or systemic diseases.

Regardless of the etiology, the nephrotic syndrome per se is associated with several clinical derangements. An eventual *decrease in plasma oncotic pressure* alters Starling forces, resulting not only in peripheral edema but ascites, pleural effusions, and a compromised intravascular volume. The latter stimulates the renin-angiotensin-aldosterone and sympathetic nervous systems, causing renal sodium retention and further aggravating the excessive accumulation of extracellular volume (see Chapter 7). Intrarenal interstitial edema and a low intravascular volume may partially explain the tendency of nephrotic individuals to develop acute renal failure.

Hyperlipidemia occurs as a result of enhanced hepatic synthesis and defective peripheral utilization of lipids, both of which are mediated by the decreased plasma oncotic pressure. Hypercholesterolemia occurs first, usually with mild hypoalbuminemia. Low-density lipoprotein (LDL) and very low-density lipoprotein (VLDL) are both elevated, whereas high-density lipoprotein (HDL) is often decreased (due to urinary loss). Hypertriglyceridemia usually occurs later and is usually associated with serum albumin concentrations of less than 2.5 g/dl. Despite the severe degree of hyperlipidemia seen in nephrotic patients, there is little to suggest a significant acceleration of atherogenesis, a point to be kept in mind when considering treatment.

Patients with nephrotic syndrome are also *hypercoagulable* owing to urinary losses of antithrombin III, protein C and protein S, venous stasis, and perhaps endothelial cell and platelet abnormalities. Not surprisingly, renal vein thrombosis (RVT) is a common occurrence with—not a cause of—the nephrotic syndrome. Membranous and membranoproliferative GN particularly seem to predispose to this complication. Although renal venography is not routinely recommended for these patients, RVT should be strongly considered in a nephrotic patient who develops pulmonary emboli, a sudden decrease in GFR, flank pain with asymmetric renal size, or a left varicocele. Softer signs of RVT include microhematuria, sterile pyuria, hyperchloremic acidosis, and variable proteinuria. In these situations, patients should undergo renal venography and if RVT is documented, receive anticoagulants for at least 3 to 6 months. The tendency for RVT to recur is well known, particularly if the nephrotic syndrome persists.

Urinary loss of various other proteins may produce abnormalities including iron deficiency *anemia* (transferrin), *low T_4 and increased T_3 resin uptake* (TBG), *osteomalacia* (25-OHD$_3$), and *immunodeficiency* (IgG and C1q).

Table 4-2 Histologic Classification, Clinical Characteristics, and Therapy of Idiopathic (Primary) Glomerulonephritis

| Disease | Microscopy | | | Clinical Presentation |
	LM	IF	EM	
Minimal-change (Nil)	"Nil"	Negative	Foot process fusion	Nephrotic
Focal segmental glomerulo-sclerosis	Focal segmental sclerosis	IgM C3 in areas of sclerosis	Subendothelial deposits; foot process fusion	Nephrotic Hypertensive
Mesangioprolifera-tive (IgM)	Focal or diffuse mesangial proliferation	Mesangial IgM, C3, IgG	Mesangial deposits	Nephrotic
Mesangioprolifera-tive (IgA) (Berger's disease)	Diffuse prolifera-tion Mesangial cells	Mesangial IgA (C3)−50% with capillary IgA	Mesangial deposits	A'Sx, gross hematuria, Nephritic
Acute Proliferative	Diffuse prolifera-tion All cells	IgG, C3 along GBM	Subepithelial de-posits− "humps"	Nephritic
Membranoprolif-erative GN	Thick BM and proliferation Duplication of BM	C3, IgG, and IgM	Mesangial, suben-dothelia de-posits (I) Intramembranous deposits (II)	Nephritic/nephrotic
Membranous GN	Thickened BM "Spike and dome"	Capillary IgG and C3	Subepithelial and intra-membranous deposits (Stages I−IV)	Nephrotic
Crescentic	Glomerular crescents	AGBM, granular IgG, or nega-tive	Variable	Nephritic RPGN
Chronic Glomerulo-sclerosis	Glomerular hyalinization and sclerosis	Variable	Variable	Chronic azo-temia, hy-pertension, proteinuria.

Table 4-2 (Continued)

Complement		Renal		Secondary
C3	C4	Mortality	Therapy	Disorders
N	N	None	Steroids	Hodgkin's disease
N	N	50% at 10 yrs.	None	Heroin, vesico-ureteral re-flux, AIDS, obesity
N	N	Unknown	Steroids (?)	
N	N	10% at 10 yrs.	None	HSP, SLE, cir-rhosis, GI pulmonary adenocar-cinomas
↓	↓	< 5% (children) < 30% (adults)	None or Antibi-otics	Post-streptococcal, SBE "shunt," visceral ab-scesses.
↓	N– ↓	40% at 10 yrs.	None or antiplate-let drugs	SLE, hepatitis B, sickle cell, neoplasia,
↓	N	60% at 10 yrs.		and others
N	N	30% at 10 yrs. 50% at 15 yrs.	Steroids Alkylating agents	SLE, hepatitis B, neoplasia, and others
N	N	High; 80% at 2 yrs.	Steroids Cytoxan, Plasmapheresis (?)	Goodpasture's, syndrome SGN, PSGN, BE, SLE, SMPGN, vasculitis
N	N	High	None	

LM = light microscopy; IF = immunofluorescence microscopy; EM = Electron microscopy; A'Sx = Asymptomatic; BM = basement membrane; RPGN = rapidly progressive glo-merulonephritis; MGN = membranous glomerulonephritis; AGBM = antiglomerular basement membrane; HSP = Henoch-Schönlein purpura; SBE = subacute bacterial endocarditis, ↓ = decreased; N = normal; N– ↓ = normal to decreased.

Table 4-3 The Clinical Classification (Syndromes) of Glomerulonephritis

Asymptomatic urinary abnormalities

Nephrotic syndrome

Nephritic syndrome

RPGN

Chronic GN

Treatment of the nephrotic syndrome should be aimed at the specific disorder, although various nonspecific treatments are also appropriate for all patients. Dietary sodium should be restricted to 250 to 500 mg daily. If edema, effusion, or ascites continue, the patient can also be given diuretics. (Cosmetic edema should be treated very conservatively.) Thiazides (hydrochlorothiazide, 25 to 50 mg, twice per day) or chlorthalidone (25 mg daily) should be tried initially. The patient can also be given triamterene, amiloride, or spironolactone for potassium sparing. One should resist the temptation to use potent loop diuretics (furosemide, bumetanide, ethacrynic acid) unless fluid retention is severe and truly refractory to sodium restriction and thiazides. Occasionally, however, severe anasarca may necessitate the use of a loop diuretic in combination with metolazone. Intravenous albumin may transiently mobilize interstitial fluid and potentiate a diuresis, but urinary protein loss ensures that this effect will be short-lived.

Determining the proper amount of dietary protein is a more difficult dilemma. Traditionally, 1.5 to 2 g of protein/kg of body weight per day has been recommended to overcome urinary protein losses and maintain plasma oncotic pressure. Recent evidence, however, suggests that serum albumin may actually increase in nephrotic patients who are on low-protein diets. This, coupled with the tendency of dietary protein to accelerate progressive nephron loss makes mild protein restriction in nephrotic patients appear more tenable. Therefore, we currently recommend a daily diet containing 0.6 g of protein/kg of body weight plus additional protein equalling urinary losses for nephrotic patients. Seventy-five percent of the dietary protein should be of high biologic value.

Nonsteroidal anti-inflammatory drugs (NSAIDs) may be useful in treating nephrotic syndrome, although considerable debate exists regarding the mechanism. Indomethacin likely decreases urinary protein loss by causing a reversible fall in GFR. Others suggest that a more specific (albeit unknown) therapeutic effect occurs with meclofenamate, particularly in focal and segmental glomerulosclerosis (FSG). The clinician must exercise extreme care when using these agents, however, since nephrotic patients are particularly prone to develop acute renal failure or other complications of the NSAID.

ACE inhibitors (captopril and enalapril) may also be useful. By decreasing intraglomerular hydrostatic pressure, these agents can cut urinary protein losses in half, particularly in diabetic nephropathy.

Ordinarily, as GFR falls, nephrotic proteinuria abates in most patients. However, with certain diseases (diabetes, amyloidosis, FSG) severe proteinuria may persist even at end-stage. In these individuals, one could consider performing a "medical nephrectomy," using mercurials or renal infarction to abolish the proteinuria and treat the nephrotic state.

Below we briefly outline the common causes of nephrotic syndrome (Table 4-4).

Table 4-4 Common Causes of the Nephrotic Syndrome

SLE

Diabetes mellitus

Amyloidosis/neoplasia

Drug use

Idiopathic (primary) glomerulopathies
    Minimal-change disease (Nil)
    Mesangioproliferative (IgM)
    FSG
    Membranous GN
    Membranoproliferative GN

Systemic Lupus Erythematosus

All patients with SLE demonstrate renal involvement on biopsy. In 40 to 90% of these patients, clinical manifestations of lupus nephritis will eventually appear, two-thirds of which will be nephrotic. However, the clinical presentation may vary considerably from mild asymptomatic hematuria and/or proteinuria to RPGN. This variability is related at least in part to the localization of immune complexes and the renal histologic pattern of lupus nephritis. The five major types of lupus nephritis and their clinical features are presented in Table 4-5 and discussed below.

Mesangioproliferative GN. Mild proliferation (in volume

Table 4-5 Histologic Varieties and Clinical Features of Lupus Nephritis

	Microscopy			
	LM	*IF*	*EM*	*Incidence*
Mesangial proliferative	Minimal mesangial proliferation	Mesangial IgG, C3	Mesangial deposits	25%
Focal proliferative	Focal and segmental proliferation of mesangial and endothial cells	Mesangial and capillary granular IgG, C3	Mesangial and capillary deposits	25%
Diffuse proliferative (DPGN)	Diffuse proliferation as above Thickened GBM (MPGN) Crescents Insterstitial nephritis	Mesangial and capillary granular IgG, C3	Mesangial and capillary deposits	25%
Membranous	Thick GBM; "spike and dome"; mesangial proliferation common	Granular IgG and C3 along GBM Occasional IgM, IgA	Subepithelial and membranous deposits	10–15%
Glomerulosclerosis	Diffuse sclerosis	Irregular IgG (IgM, IgA) deposition	Sclerosis	10%

and number) of mesangial cells may be the initial stage of renal involvement in SLE. Approximately 25% of patients with clinically detectable disease will have this histologic pattern, usually with asymptomatic hematuria and proteinuria and occasionally with nephrotic syndrome. Mesangial localization of IgG and complement (C3) are common; serum complements may be normal or decreased. Although the prognosis is good for renal survival, mesangioproliferative GN may progress to a more aggressive lesion.

Focal Proliferative GN. These patients are usually nephritic, occasionally nephrotic, with well-preserved renal function. Progression to the diffuse proliferative lesion is quite common. In fact, "severe" forms of this lesion have a prognosis not unlike that of

Table 4-5 (Continued)

Clinical Syndrome	Complement		Renal Mortality	Therapy for Renal Disease	Comments
	C3	C4			
Mild Asymptomatic	N−↓	N−↓	Slight, but may progress	None	
Nephritic, rarely nephrotic	N−↓	N−↓	30% at 10 yrs.	Daily or alternate day steroids	Can progress to DPGN "Severe" forms have prognosis similar to DPGN
Nephritic, nephrotic, RPGN	↓	N−↓	80% at 10 yrs.	"Pulse" & oral steroids; "Pulse" cyclophosphamide	"Chronicity" index may predict outcome and guide therapy
Nephrotic	N−↓	N	20% at 5 yrs. 30−50% at 10 yrs.	Alternate day steroids (?)	
Chronic azotemia Hypertension Proteinuria	N	N			

LM = Light microscopy; IF = Immunofluorescene microscopy; EM = Electron microscopy; N = normal; N−↓ = normal to decreased.

diffuse proliferative GN. IgG and C3 deposits are usually identified in mesangial and subendothelial locations. Occasionally, segmental crescents can be identified.

Diffuse Proliferative GN. This lesion is most common in patients with lupus nephritis who progress to end-stage renal failure. Microscopy shows diffuse proliferation, usually with crescents. A rapidly progressive clinical picture often occurs. Thickening of the basement membrane may produce a membranoproliferative histologic picture. Variable degrees of interstitial inflammation and fibrosis are also common. Histologic indices (Activity Index, Chronicity Index) aid in predicting outcome and perhaps also in determining therapy with cytotoxic agents for patients with this lesion.

Membranous GN. Histologically and clinically, membranous lupus nephritis differs little from idiopathic membranous GN (see below).

Glomerulosclerosis. Advanced scarring of most glomeruli occurs with this lesion, which likely represents the end result of both membranous and proliferative forms of lupus nephritis. Arteriolar and interstitial scarring are also common. Most patients have significant azotemia at this point in the course of the diseases and eventually require renal replacement therapy.

Although division of lupus nephritis into distinct categories may be helpful conceptually, prognostically, and therapeutically, the clinician must always remember that tremendous clinical and histologic overlap often occurs, making strict classification sometimes misleading. Lupus nephritis is a dynamic process and may progress or regress, depending not only on the localization of immune complexes but also on a variety of other factors, including patient age, hypertension, medications (analgesics, NSAIDs), and perhaps diet. Treatment should therefore be aimed at delaying or preventing the progression of renal disease in those patients at greatest risk, and not at a specific histology or laboratory feature.

Treatment of lupus nephritis is extremely controversial. Steroids are a well-accepted mainstay. Other immunosuppressives (chlorambucil, nitrogen mustard, azathioprine [Imuran], cyclophosphamide) have been used for years in both controlled and uncontrolled settings. Although they occasionally seem beneficial, controlled trials have usually failed to demonstrate unequivocal benefit. When data from several studies are pooled, immunosuppressive therapy plus steroids may be better than treatment with steroids alone, but it is also associated with a higher risk. One exception appears to be the use of "pulse" cyclophosphamide (0.5 to 1.0 g/m^2 body surface area [BSA]). Given monthly, this treatment produces excellent subjective and objective improvement while allowing a reduction in steroid dosage.

A recent controlled clinical trial of plasmapheresis concluded that it had no beneficial effect on the clinical, renal, or serologic course of patients with lupus nephritis. Its use in treating lupus nephritis should therefore be abandoned.

Efficacy of treatment can be judged by repeat renal biopsy (rarely necessary), changes in renal function or urine sediment and a variety of serologic markers of disease activity including anti-DNA, C3, C4, and assays of circulating immune complexes.

Diabetic Nephropathy

Diabetic nephropathy is the most common cause of nephrotic syndrome in adults. Forty to sixty percent of all insulin-dependent diabetics will eventually develop this complication of diabetes mellitus, usually after 12 to 15 years. Coincident with or shortly after the onset of nephrosis, diabetics usually develop progressive azotemia and hypertension. End-stage renal disease typically occurs within 2 to 5 years, and death, regardless of therapy, usually follows within another 1 to 5 years. Figure 4-1 outlines this natural history and attempts to correlate the clinical features with glomerular structural changes.

Glomerulosclerosis is invariably seen on light microscopy associated with the nephrotic syndrome. This may be either global and diffuse or nodular (Kimmelstiel-Wilson syndrome). Both lesions can be found on most biopsies. Often, both afferent and efferent arterioles are hyalinized, a feature unique to diabetic nephropathy. Although fluorescence microscopy is usually negative, it may show nonspecific linear staining for IgG (and albumin) along the base-

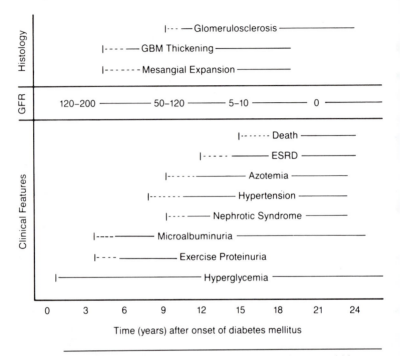

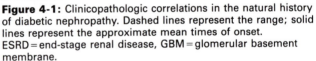

Figure 4-1: Clinicopathologic correlations in the natural history of diabetic nephropathy. Dashed lines represent the range; solid lines represent the approximate mean times of onset.
ESRD = end-stage renal disease, GBM = glomerular basement membrane.

ment membranes. Electron microscopy shows thickened basement membranes and an increase in mesangial volume.

Once these histolopathologic changes (and nephrotic syndrome) have appeared, there is nothing one can do to reverse the disease and little one can do to alter the rate of progressive deterioration. Strict glucose control has little effect on the disease. ACE inhibitors (captopril, enalapril) will decrease urinary protein losses. Control of systemic hypertension will delay but not prevent end-stage renal failure. Decreasing intraglomerular hypertension with angiotensin-converting enzyme inhibitors and a protein-restricted diet may similarly slow (but not abrogate) the progressive loss of function. It therefore appears that for any therapy to have a significant impact on the natural history of diabetic nephropathy, it will need to be initiated before the onset of nephrosis.

Early in the course of diabetes, three features may appear (see Fig. 4-1): (1) excretion of small quantities of albumin (microalbuminuria and exercise-induced albuminuria), (2) an increased GFR (hyperfiltration) perhaps caused by hyperglycemia, and (3) abnormal histology, including thickening of the basement membrane and mesangial expansion. Of these, both microalbuminuria and hyperfiltration appear to be early markers for the eventual occurrence of clinical diabetic nephropathy. Whether these abnormalities are pathogenetically related to nephrotic syndrome is still under debate. However, recent studies in animals strongly suggest that the early hyperfiltration seen in many diabetics is a proximate cause of microalbuminuria, damage to the glomerular basement membrane (GBM) with eventual glomerulosclerosis, and its consequent clinical manifestations. This hyperfiltration theory must therefore be included with the metabolic theory (i.e., lack of insulin and hyperglycemia effect changes in the glomerulus) and basement membrane theory (i.e., abnormalities are genetically determined) when considering the pathogenesis and treatment of diabetic nephropathy.

If intraglomerular hypertension and hyperfiltration indeed prove to be responsible for diabetic nephropathy, one could certainly envision strict glucose control and angiotensin II inhibitors (to lower intraglomerular hydrostatic pressure) to be of benefit early in the course of the disease. Historically, glucose control has correlated poorly with the development of nephrotic syndrome. Studies are currently underway to evaluate the early use of angiotensin-converting enzyme inhibitors. Identification and early treatment of those diabetics with elevated GFR and microalbuminuria may well be the standard of care within the next few years.

Several other clinical features of diabetic nephropathy are noteworthy. Although present in only 25% of patients with diabetic nephropathy initially, hypertension eventually develops in most. Microhematuria (without RBC casts) is common, occurring in 30 to

50 percent. The kidneys are normal to large in size, despite severe azotemia. Retinopathy strongly correlates with the presence of nephropathy (as do peripheral and autonomic neuropathy, albeit less so). Hyperkalemia and hyporeninemic hypoaldosteronism are also commonly seen. This constellation of findings is so unique with nephrotic syndrome that a renal biopsy is rarely necessary to confirm the diagnosis of diabetic nephropathy.

Amyloidosis/Neoplasia

Amyloidosis (mean age of 60 to 65 years) should be considered in all elderly patients with nephrotic syndrome. Renal involvement occurs in 75% of these patients, half of whom are nephrotic. Kidney size is enlarged symmetrically. The renal disease is progressive, resulting in renal failure over a period of months to years (5-year survival rate of 20%). In most patients, monoclonal proteins can be identified in the serum or urine sometime during the clinical course.

The glomerular disease results from the deposition of insoluble polypeptide aggregates derived from either a portion of immunoglobulin light-chains or some other byproduct of chronic inflammation. The deposits are identified by 80 to 100 Å fibrils seen by electron microscopy and as amorphous material in the mesangium; they are occasionally identified as capillary loops (resembling diabetic nephropathy) by light microscopy, particularly on staining with congo red. Blood vessels are also commonly involved, making percutaneous renal biopsy somewhat precarious in these patients.

Neoplasia may account for 5 to 15% of cases of otherwise idiopathic nephrotic syndrome, necessitating that strong consideration be given to this possibility, particularly in elderly patients. Patients with carcinomas, lymphomas, Hodgkin's disease, and myeloma may all present with nephrosis. The common histologic lesions associated with neoplasms are listed in Table 4-6.

The nephrotic syndrome will usually antedate or coincide with the malignancy with approximately equal frequency. The pathogenesis appears related to antibody formation against various tumor

Table 4-6 Neoplasia-Associated Nephrotic Syndrome

Incidence	Lesion	Neoplasia
70%	Membranous	Carcinoma (lung, breast, colon, kidney, stomach, cervix, and others) Lymphoma

10%	Membrano-
	    proliferative
		Carcinoma
		Occasionally lymphoma and leukemias
		    with/without cryoglobulinemia

5–10%	Minimal-change	Hodgkin's disease Lymphoma (occasionally) Carcinoma (rarely)
5%	Amyloidosis	Carcinoma Multiple myeloma Lymphoma
<5%	Crescentic	Carcinoma Lymphoma
<5%	FSG	Carcinoma

antigens (circulating or in situ). Direct deposition of amyloid may also occur.

When considering neoplasms and nephrosis, one should remember the entire spectrum of renal disease associated with malignancy, including obstruction, tumor lysis syndrome, uric acid nephropathy, hypercalcemia, hyperviscosity, and light-chain nephropathy.

Drugs

Numerous drugs are associated with the nephrotic syndrome (Table 4-7). Membranous GN with typical granular IgG deposits is a characteristic result of penicillamine, captopril (in high dosages), and gold therapy suggesting an immune complex pathogenesis. A particularly malignant form of focal glomerulosclerosis appears to be related to heroin and amphetamine use. NSAIDs (particularly fenoprofen) induce a minimal change lesion, often associated with variable degrees of acute interstitial inflammation and ARF.

Table 4-7 Drug-Induced Nephrotic Syndrome

Lesion	Drug
Membranous	Penicillamine
	Captopril
	Gold
	Mercury
FSG	Heroin
	Amphetamines
Minimal-change	Nonsteroidals
	Fenoprofen
	Ibuprofen
	Indomethacin
	Naproxen
	Sulindac
	Tolmetin

Idiopathic (Primary) Nephrotic Syndrome

If no obvious cause is identified, patients with nephrotic syndrome are usually classified as idiopathic. Any one of several primary renal diseases (as defined by light microscopy) may be responsible. These are briefly discussed below and outlined in Table 4-2.

Minimal Change Disease. Minimal change disease (Nil disease, lipoid nephrosis) is the most common cause of nephrotic syndrome in children (80%) and is responsible for 10 to 15% of cases of nephrotic syndrome in adults. The clinical presentation is that of pure nephrotic syndrome, although microhematuria, hypertension, and azotemia may rarely occur, particularly in adults. Patients often have an atopic history (urticaria, asthma). Serum IgG may be decreased; immunoglobulin M(IgM) may be elevated. Serum complement levels are normal. Light microscopy generally shows no abnormalities, immunofluorescence is negative, and electron microscopy shows "fusion" of epithelial cell foot processes.

Patients generally run a benign clinical course, suffering some morbidity of the nephrotic syndrome per se but virtually no renal mortality. Spontaneous remission and relapse are common. Minimal change disease is highly sensitive to treatment with corticosteroids, but in view of the excellent natural history, steroids should be reserved for those patients with significant morbidity from the nephrotic syndrome. For the patient who commonly suffers relapse or for the rare, steroid-resistant patient, short courses of chlorambucil or cytoxan (but not Imuran) have been used successfully.

Although the pathogenesis of minimal change disease is unknown, several factors point to an immunologic (perhaps cell-mediated) mechanism, including (1) its frequency in atopic individuals, (2) its extreme steroid sensitivity, (3) its association with Hodgkin's disease, (4) its association with an increased prevalence of HLA-B12, and (5) the release of a lymphokine-like factor by cultured lymphocytes of patients with this lesion. In addition, minimal change disease, mesangioproliferative (IgM) GN, and idiopathic focal segmental glomerulosclerosis (FSG) may all exist as a spectrum of the same disease process.

Focal Segmental Glomerulosclerosis. FSG (focal sclerosis) accounts for 10 to 15% of cases of idiopathic nephrotic syndrome in children and adults. It carries a far more serious prognosis than minimal change disease. Hematuria and hypertension may occur in 30 to 50% of patients, and progressive loss of renal function is the rule. Although spontaneous complete remission is reported (usually in children), the 10-year renal mortality rate is 50%. Approximately 20% of patients run a more "malignant" course, with renal failure occurring within 2 to 5 years. The disease is resistant to corticosteroids and there is little to support the use of cytotoxic therapy. Meclofenamate may be of some help. FSG recurs in patients who have undergone renal transplants, recurring more frequently in those with the more aggressive pretransplant disease.

Light microscopy reveals sclerosis in some areas (segmental) of some glomeruli (focal). The process may begin in the deeper juxtamedullary glomeruli, making sampling error a constant problem. In the areas of sclerosis, fluorescence microscopy reveals IgM and C3 in a granular fashion. Serum IgG, IgM, and C3 are normal. Electron microscopy demonstrates diffuse foot process fusion (reminiscent of minimal change disease) and electron-dense amorphous material (usually in the subendothelial location) adjacent to sclerotic areas.

In its idiopathic form, FSG is likely the end result of a disease spectrum that includes minimal change disease and mesangioproliferative (IgM) GN. It is also the glomerulopathy noted with such diverse renal insults as vesicoureteral reflux, heroin abuse, and analgesic nephropathy. In the experimental "remnant kidney" model of progressive renal failure, FSG is universal. In addition, this lesion is commonly found when nephrotic syndrome complicates acquired immunodeficiency syndrome (AIDS) and obesity. FSG therefore appears to be the common histologic result of a heterogenous group of renal insults causing constant and unrelenting proteinuria. The constant fluorescence finding of IgM in FSG may thus be a nonspecific consequence of continual macromolecular filtration.

Mesangioproliferative GN. Although patients with mesangioproliferative (IgM) GN usually present with the nephrotic syndrome, non-nephrotic proteinuria is also commonly seen. As with FSG, hypertension and hematuria may be seen in as many as 30% of cases, but unlike patients with FSG, those with mesangioproliferative GN frequently undergo spontaneous remission. Success with steroid and cytotoxic therapy is less than with minimal change disease, but greater than with FSG. When there is no remission, the disease often progresses to FSG and may be an intermediate lesion between minimal change disease and FSG.

Light microscopy shows an increase in the number and volume of mesangial cells. Mesangial IgM and C3 can usually be demonstrated by fluorescence microscopy. Electron microscopy usually shows electron-dense material in the mesangium, as well. The pathogenesis of mesangioproliferative GN is unknown, and its prognosis is uncertain.

Membranous GN. Membranous GN (MGN) is commonly seen in adults with idiopathic nephrotic syndrome (30 to 40%), but rarely in children. Besides its idiopathic variety, MGN is commonly associated with a wide variety of other diseases including SLE, hepatitis B infection, carcinomas, and non-Hodgkin's lymphomas (Table 4-8). These secondary causes should always be considered in patients with otherwise idiopathic MGN.

MGN progresses more slowly than FSG. At 10 years, 30 to 50% of patients will be at end-stage, but as many as 70% may ultimately

Table 4-8 Systemic (Secondary) Causes of Membranous and Membranoproliferative Glomerulonephritis

	MGN	*MPGN*
Immune	SLE Mixed connective tissue disease Sjögren's syndrome	SLE Mixed connective tissue disease Cryoglobulinemia
Toxins	Gold Mercury Penicillamine ?(Captopril) Primidone	
Infections	Hepatitis B Treponema Malaria Schistosomiasis	Hepatitis B Bacterial endocarditis Visceral sepsis Shunt nephritis Malaria Syphilis
Neoplasm	Carcinomas (many) Lymphoma	Carcinomas
Other	Thyroiditis	Sickle cell disease Hereditary C2 deficiency

progress if followed longer. Spontaneous partial and complete remission may occur in an additional 30%, making interpretation of therapeutic studies difficult. Nevertheless, controlled clinical trials with alternate day steroids alone and combinations of "pulse" and oral steroids with chlorambucil suggest that the progression to end-stage renal failure in MGN can be slowed and perhaps prevented.

Although MGN appears to be immune complex mediated, considerable debate exists regarding circulating or in situ complex formation. Electron microscopy demonstrates a progression (roughly correlating to clinical severity) of electron-dense deposits from the subepithelial (Stage I) to intramembranous (Stage IV) locations. Staining (with silver methenamine) of normal basement membrane material around these deposits demonstrates the characteristic "spike and dome" pattern as well as diffuse basement membrane thickening by light microscopy. Immunofluorescence shows granular deposition of IgG and C3 along the basement membrane.

Membranoproliferative GN. Membranoproliferative GN (mesangiocapillary GN, hypocomplementemic GN, MPGN) is usually seen in children or young adults and often appears to be hereditary. Most patients present with nephrotic syndrome, although hematuria (often macroscopic) is also very common, as is hypertension and azotemia. Hence, MPGN is often termed the nephritic/nephrotic disease.

There appear to be at least two distinct types (Type I and Type II) of MPGN. Although both types have similar clinical presentations, they seem to have a very different pathogenesis. Type I appears to be immune complex–mediated as evidenced by diffuse granular deposition of IgG or IgM and C3 along the GBM by immunofluorescence. In addition, electron-dense deposits regularly appear in subendothelial and mesangial locations on electron microscopy. Light microscopy shows diffuse proliferation of mesangial cells and an increase in mesangial matrix, which appears to "intrude" and separate the basement membrane, producing a "tram track" appearance. This microscopic appearance is commonly seen in a variety of infections (see Table 4-8), including bacterial endocarditis, visceral sepsis, and hepatitis B. All are believed to be of immune complex pathogenesis and all must be diligently excluded whenever Type I MPGN is documented.

Type II MPGN (dense-deposit disease) is a fascinating, usually idiopathic disorder associated with continual activation of the alternate complement pathway by a circulating autoantibody, C3 Nephritic Factor (C3 NeF). Serum C3 is therefore nearly uniformly decreased, whereas C4 may be normal. Although on light microscopy, Type II resembles Type I, dense intramembranous deposits are evident by electron microscopy.

Both types are indolently progressive, and spontaneous remissions are uncommon. Therapeutically, steroids are disappointing and alkylating agents of no benefit. Antiplatelet therapy may be of some use in slowing the progression to end-stage renal failure that occurs in 40 to 80% of patients with MPGN. In patients who undergo renal transplants, recurrence of Type II MPGN should be expected. Recurrence of Type I disease is less common.

Nephritic Syndrome

The nephritic syndrome is the constellation of hematuria with RBC casts, modest proteinuria (generally less than 2.5 g/day) and variable degrees of oliguria, azotemia, and hypertension. Circulatory congestion with edema is also commonly seen. In general, this syndrome reflects a more fulminant inflammation of the glomerulus. Because of its more fulminant nature, nephritic patients are often hypocomplementemic, which may be useful in differential diagnosis.

Table 4-9 lists the common causes of nephritic syndrome. Table 4-10 classifies these according to serum complement.

Table 4-9 Common Causes of the Nephritic Syndrome

Systemic lupus erythematosus

Infectious GN
  Post-streptococcal GN
  Bacterial endocarditis
  Shunt nephritis
  Visceral abscess
  Hepatitis B antigenemia

Vasculitis
  Polyarteritis nodosa
  Wegener's granulomatosis
  Hypersensitivity vasculitis
  Cryoglobulinemia
  Henoch-Schönlein purpura

Hereditary nephritis (Alport's syndrome)

Idiopathic (primary) glomerulopathies
  Acute proliferative GN
  Mesangioproliferative (IgA) GN (Berger's disease)
  Membranoproliferative GN

Table 4-10 Classification of Nephritic Syndrome Based on Serum Complement*

	Low C3	Normal C3
Secondary GN	Lupus nephritis (70–90%)	Polyarteritis nodosa
	Bacterial endocarditis (90%)	Hypersensitivity vasculitis
	"Shunt" nephritis (90%)	Wegener's syndrome
	Cryoglobulinemia (85%)	Henoch-Schönlein purpura
		Goodpasture's syndrome
Primary GN	Post-streptococcal GN (90%)	Berger's (IgA) nephropathy
	MPGN	RPGN
	Type I (60–80%)	Idiopathic GN
	Type II (90%)	AGBM
		Immune complex
		No immune deposits

* Percentages indicate the approximate frequencies of depressed C3.

Systemic Lupus Erythematosus

Lupus nephritis frequently presents with a nephritic syndrome, particularly with the proliferative lesions. Hypocomplementia can be expected in these patients.

Infectious GN

Numerous infections are associated with active GN producing the nephritic syndrome. With post-streptococcal GN (PSGN), the nephritic syndrome usually follows a 1- to 3-week latent period. Treatment with antibiotics is ineffectual. With other infectious glomerulopathies, the nephritis is coincident with the infection and resolves with antibiotic therapy. Examples of these include bacterial endocarditis, "shunt nephritis," occult visceral abscess hepatitis B antigenemia, *Klebsiella* and pneumococcal pneumonias, and a variety of other bacterial, viral, and parasitic diseases.

Sixty to 80% of patients with bacterial endocarditis will have nephritis. In addition to the usual clinical features of endocarditis, a positive rheumatoid factor, hypocomplementemia (C3 and C4), and increased levels of circulating immune complexes are usually documented. Similar serologic studies are seen with infected ventricular-atrial shunts ("shunt nephritis") and with occult intra-abdominal or pulmonary abscesses with septicemia.

Acute GN and hypocomplementemia may also accompany hepatitis B antigenemia either acutely or with the chronic carrier state, where it is seen without overt hepatic disease. Many of these patients have cryoimmunoglobulinemia with a clinical syndrome of vasculitis and purpura.

As one might expect, these diseases present a spectrum of histologic findings. Light microscopy shows a proliferative lesion that may be focal or diffuse, with or without crescents. A membranoproliferative lesion is also commonly encountered, particularly with hepatitis B. Immunofluorescence microscopy shows granular deposition of IgG (and occasionally IgM) and C3 along the GBM and in the mesangium. Deposits are invariably seen in the subendothelial space.

Vasculitis

Systemic vasculitis is a common cause of the nephritic syndrome, and includes polyarteritis nodosa (and associated overlap syndromes), Wegener's granulomatosis, hypersensitivity vasculitis, Henoch-Schönlein purpura, and cryoglobulinemia. The hemolytic-uremic syndromes (HUS/TTP) may also present with nephritic syndrome. These syndromes are outlined in detail in Chapter 6.

Hereditary Nephritis and Alport's syndrome

A clinical spectrum of hereditary glomerulopathies exists. At one end is the syndrome of benign familial hematuria (see Chapter 2), with which affected patients have isolated microscopic hematuria and irregular thinning of the GBM. At the other extreme are patients with progressive renal failure. Alport's syndrome refers to those patients with nephritis and a bilateral sensorineural hearing deficit. Hereditary nephritis refers to those patients without hearing defects. Both groups of patients may have various other features, including ocular abnormalities (particularly those of the lens) and thrombocytopenia with giant platelets. In addition, irregular thickening and splitting of the GBM is usually observed in both.

The clinical syndrome of microhematuria, RBC casts, variable proteinuria, and progressive azotemia (often progressing to end-stage renal disease [ESRD] between the ages of 20 and 40 years) affects males more often than females. Affected females have less obvious urinary abnormalities and rarely develop uremia. These differences appear related to the X-linked dominant pattern of inheritance with variable expression in women.

Most investigators agree that the incidence of hereditary nephritis is underestimated and that many cases go unrecognized. Careful attention to family history as well as a historical and audiometric search for hearing-loss should help identify this cause of the nephritic syndrome.

Idiopathic (Primary) Nephritic Syndrome

If no obvious cause is identified, patients with the nephritic syndrome are usually classified as idiopathic. Three primary renal diseases (defined by light microscopy) should be considered in this situation. These are discussed below and outlined in Table 4-2.

Acute Proliferative GN. This can be seen with or without a recent streptococcal infection, although PSGN is the prototype of this disease. It is characterized by the abrupt onset of hematuria, edema, hypertension, and azotemia 1 to 2 weeks after an acute Group A, beta-hemolytic streptococcal infection, 50% or more of which are cutaneous. Specific antibodies to streptococcal antigens are usually identifiable in these patients and include antistreptolysin-O (ASO) (rarely with cutaneous infections), antistreptokinase (ASK), anti-DNAse B and antihyaluronidase. Most laboratories will offer a screening battery (Streptozyme Panel, Wampole).

Histologically, a diffuse proliferation of all cells (mesangial, endothelial, epithelial, and polys) is seen by light microscopy (Table 4-2). Immunofluorescence demonstrates granular deposition of IgG and C3 along the GBM and in the mesangium. Characteristic subepithelial "humps" of immune deposits are seen by light microscopy.

The pathogenesis is immune complex mediated, most likely with in situ binding of antibody to a foreign antigen (or altered native antigen) on the epithelial side of the GBM. Subsequent activation of the complement system (in part via the alternate pathway) mediates the inflammatory response. Serum complement (C3) falls transiently, returning to baseline within 3 to 6 months.

Although most patients with PSGN are nephritic, a wide spectrum of clinical findings may be present—from asymptomatic hematuria to RPGN with glomerular crescents. Except in these rare cases of RPGN, the prognosis for renal recovery is excellent; 95% of children and at least 60 to 70% of adults usually experience recovery. Slow progression (i.e., progression over a period of years) to chronic proteinuria, hypertension, and/or end-stage renal failure does occur, usually in adults. Treatment of the acute illness is supportive. Antibiotics are not indicated unless active strep infection persists (or in other types of infectious GN discussed above). Corticosteroids are ineffective.

Mesangioproliferative (IgA) GN. Mesangioproliferative GN (Berger's disease, IgA nephropathy) is a disease characterized by microscopic hematuria with recurrent macroscopic hematuria, and which usually develops in children and young adults. Episodes of gross hematuria usually coincide with a brief viral upper respiratory or gastrointestinal illness. Although asymptomatic hematuria is the most common, a host of other clinical aberrancies may occur, such as nephrotic syndrome (5 to 15%), acute nephritic syndrome, and (rarely) RPGN.

IgA nephropathy is as heterogeneous pathologically as it is clinically. Light microscopy may show minimal changes or necrotizing and crescentic lesions, although mild mesangial proliferation is the rule. IgA deposition in mesangial cells is universal. Occasionally, IgG, IgM, and C3 may also be found. Electron-dense deposits are usual in the mesangium, but are rarely seen in subendothelial areas.

The wide range of clinical and histologic features probably reflects a variable pathogenesis related to overproduction or decreased clearance of IgA. Fifty percent of patients have an elevated serum IgA. Circulating immune complexes cannot be identified by usual methods. Mesangial deposits of IgA are also seen with a variety of other disorders, including Henoch-Schönlein purpura, SLE, cirrhosis, pulmonary or gastrointestinal mucin-secreting adenocarcinomas, and ankylosing spondylitis.

The prognosis is generally excellent. However, 10 to 15 percent may follow a more aggressive course to renal failure over a period of 10 to 15 years. Proteinuria and hypertension correlate with a poor prognosis. Renal function may also transiently deteriorate coincident with episodes of gross hematuria. No treatment is known to be effective.

Membranoproliferative GN. MPGN is usually a nephrotic disease, although patients may have nephritic signs, as well, such as hematuria, RBC casts, hypertension, and azotemia. This nephritic/nephrotic syndrome is particularly common with the systemic disorders associated with MPGN (see Table 4-8), particularly SLE and bacterial infections.

Rapidly Progressive Glomerulonephritis

RPGN is a clinical syndrome that may occur with several different diseases. Its most common feature is a rapid deterioration of renal function. Most patients experience at least a doubling of serum creatinine over 3 months, with progression to end-stage renal failure over a period of weeks to months. Other clinical findings may variably include hematuria, RBC casts, proteinuria (occasionally nephrotic), and hypertension. Renal size is usually well-preserved. Patients are generally older (mean age of 50 to 60 years in most series).

Glomerular crescent formation is a nearly uniform finding in patients with RPGN, regardless of etiology. Thus RPGN and "crescentic" GN have become synonymous, even though crescents may often be seen histologically in patients without a fulminant clinical course. Light microscopy also shows focal or diffuse proliferation with necrosis of glomerular capillaries. Focal disruption of the GBM are also seen by electron microscopy. Depending on the etiology, immunofluorescence may either show granular immune complex deposition, linear-staining AGBM antibody, or no immune deposits.

Table 4-11 outlines the common causes of RPGN. The "nephritic" group of diseases, including postinfectious GN (e.g., PSGN), IgA nephropathy, MPGN, and SLE account for about 15% of all cases.

Systemic vasculitis (outlined in Chapter 6) accounts for an additional 15% of cases. Patients with systemic vasculitis may or may not demonstrate immune complex deposition on renal biopsy.

Goodpasture's disease is the clinical triad of pulmonary hemorrhage, GN, and circulating AGBM antibody. The antibody (usually IgG) can be detected by radioimmunoassay or linear staining along the GBM on renal biopsy. Cross reactivity of the antibody with the alveolar capillary basement membrane (also demonstrable by immunofluorescence) produces alveolitis and the pulmonary hemor-

Table 4-11 Common Causes of Rapidly Progressive Glomerulonephritis*

Nephritis group (15%)
    Acute proliferative
    IgA nephropathy
    MPGN
    Infectious GN
    SLE

Vasculitis group (15%)
    Polyarteritis
    Wegener's syndrome
    Hypersensitivity
    Henoch-Schönlein purpura
    Cryoglobulinemia

Goodpasture's syndrome (15%)

Idiopathic GN (60%)
    AGBM
    Immune complex
    No immune deposits

*Percentages represent approximate frequencies.

rhage. Previously damaged alveoli are apparently necessary to produce the pulmonary hemorrhage; hence, Goodpasture's is a disease almost exclusively of smokers.

Young males are most often affected, with the hemoptysis usually preceding the nephritis. Both the pulmonary and renal manifestations may vary from mild to severe. Hypertension is usually absent. Serum complement is normal. Goodpasture's disease accounts for approximately 15% of cases of RPGN.

Sixty percent of cases of RPGN are *idiopathic*. By fluorescence microscopy they are evenly divided into those with the AGBM antibody (without Goodpasture's disease) (one-third), granular immune complex deposition (one-third), and no immune deposits (one-third). This latter category of a rapidly progressive clinical course and glomerular crescents without immune deposits is believed by some to be a vasculitis confined only to the kidney. Some may have an antineutrophilic cytoplasmic antibody identified in the plasma. The term "limited Wegener's" is often used to describe this condition.

For all forms of RPGN left untreated, the prognosis is extremely poor. This, coupled with the success of recent therapies necessitates an aggressive diagnostic approach with early renal biopsy for patients with RPGN. Pulse methylprednisolone therapy is generally accepted as efficacious for most patients, although treatment with pulse steroids alone is not adequate for patients with Goodpasture's disease. For these patients, uncontrolled trials using plasmapheresis and immunosuppressive drugs, particularly oral or pulse cyclophosphamide, have had dramatic results. Not unexpectedly, the response to plasmapheresis is less favorable for patients in whom immune deposits are not identified (approximately one-fourth to one-third of all patients with RPGN).

Chronic Glomerulonephritis

All of the previously described glomerulopathies can progress to a chronic form. Indeed, chronic GN is believed to be the potential "final common pathway" for most diseases primarily affecting the glomerulus. However, at least one-third of patients will have no known previous history of glomerulonephritis or other urinary abnormality.

Except for RPGN, there is generally a slow and insidious progression toward ESRD. In addition to azotemia, patients usually have anemia, hypertension, and proteinuria. The degree of proteinuria is usually less than nephrotic-range and decreases as GFR falls (except in patients with amyloid, diabetic nephropathy, or FSG, whose nephrotic syndrome often persists despite ESRD). Broad casts are typically seen on urinalysis. Small symmetrically contracted kidneys are the rule.

Renal histology similarly reflects an indolent progression with glomerular sclerosis and hyalinization, although active inflammation and proliferation may occasionally persist. Tubules are atrophied and arteriolar sclerosis is common, as is chronic interstitial inflammation and fibrosis. As individual diseases merge into this common histologic pattern, a specific diagnosis is extremely difficult to make. Similarly, once the serum creatinine is more than 6 mg/dl and/or renal size is less than 8.5 to 9 cm, specific therapy is nearly impossible. The utility of the renal biopsy is therefore significantly compromised and is rarely helpful in these patients.

Diagnostic Approach

The approach to patients with glomerular disease involves three major steps:

1. Considering the possibility of glomerular disease.
2. Considering the five major clinical syndromes of GN and determining which best categorizes the patient.
3. Considering the specific diagnoses of nephrotic syndrome, nephritic syndrome, and RPGN.

Figure 4-2 demonstrates the criteria necessary to make a diagnosis of glomerular disease in a patient with an isolated abnormality (e.g., hematuria, proteinuria). In most patients, a thoughtful

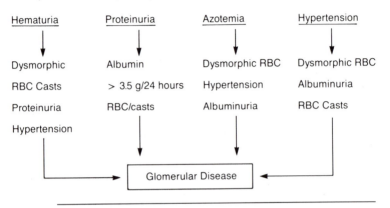

Figure 4-2: Diagnostic approach to glomerular disease (Step 1). The typical signs of glomerular dysfunction are identified.

examination of the urine sediment and quantitation of urinary protein are sufficient. (This evaluation is more completely delineated in Chapter 2.)

Next, one should categorize the patient into one of the major clinical syndromes of GN. Figure 4-3 schematically demonstrates

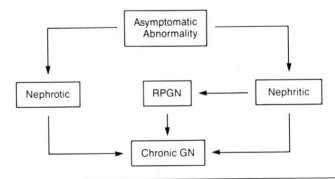

Figure 4-3: Diagnostic approach to glomerular disease (Step 2). The five major clinical syndromes of GN are considered.

these major syndromes and their interrelationships. The arrows represent probable progression and perhaps remission of these disorders. Although not clearly represented here, a patient can develop chronic GN without an antecedent history of nephrosis, (e.g., RPGN). In fact, conceptually, the individual diseases comprising nephrotic syndrome, nephritic syndrome, or RPGN can present with chronic GN, or if milder, with an asymptomatic abnormality.

One must also remember that the syndromes outlined here are not mutually exclusive. Individual diseases distinctly classified here as nephrotic, nephritic, or RPGN may not be so distinct clinically. For example, the vasculitides, here classified with nephritic syndrome or RPGN, may occasionally present as pure nephrotic syndrome. *Because of this clinical overlap, one should always consider the differential diagnosis of each major syndrome in every patient.*

Figures 4-4 to 4-6 outline a diagnostic and therapeutic approach

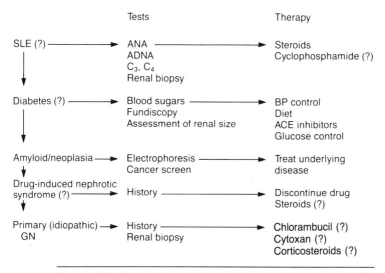

Figure 4-4: Diagnostic approach to glomerular disease (Step 3). Diagnostic and therapeutic approach to the nephrotic syndrome. BP = blood pressure; ACE = angiotensin-converting enzyme.

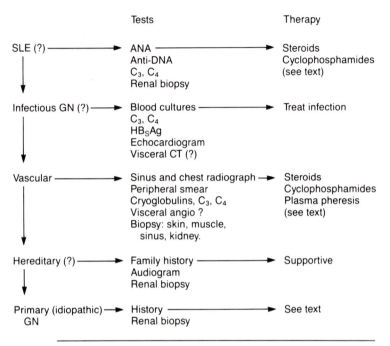

Figure 4-5: Diagnostic approach to glomerular disease (Step 3). Diagnostic and therapeutic approach to the nephritic syndrome.

to nephrotic syndrome, nephritic syndrome, and RPGN, respectively. The tests that are necessary to support or confirm a diagnosis are also listed. For nephrotic syndrome, a renal biopsy is not absolutely necessary. However, except in the case of diabetic nephropathy where renal biopsy contributes little, there are usually enough differences regarding therapy of these diseases to make the biopsy helpful.

For all patients with nephritic syndrome, blood cultures, serologic screening, and hepatitis B surface antigen (HB$_s$Ag) are important. If vasculitis is a strong consideration, visceral angiography and skin or skeletal muscle biopsy should be considered first. Often the renal biopsy is nonspecific in these patients.

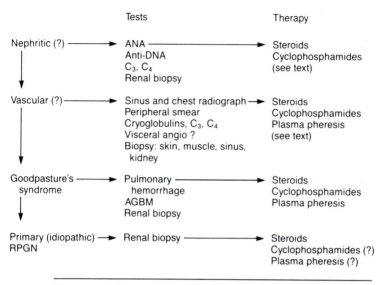

Figure 4-6: Diagnostic approach to glomerular disease (Step 3). Diagnostic and therapeutic approach to RPGN.

An aggressive approach including early renal biopsy is mandatory for all patients with RPGN. Effective therapies are available, and the patient's condition may otherwise deteriorate very quickly. Prompt diagnosis and treatment are therefore essential.

Case 4-1: *Discussion*

1. The triad of massive proteinuria (>3.5 g/24 hr), edema, and hypoalbuminemia confirm that this patient has nephrotic syndrome.

Numerous diagnostic possibilities exist (see Fig. 4-4). First, the patient does have diabetes requiring medication. The absence of diabetic retinopathy (excluded by fluorescein angiography) makes this diagnosis suspect, however.

ANA, Anti-DNA, C3 and C4 were all normal, essentially excluding SLE. In this patient, general physical examination revealed the presence of a thyroid nodule. This is of concern because occult neoplasia is often associated with nephrotic syndrome (usually with MGN) in patients older than 50 years of age (see Table 4-6). Alternatively, the combination of nephrotic syndrome and azotemia make FSG likely. This is particularly true in view of the patient's previous history of nephrectomy, which appears to predispose to this lesion, and his body weight, since FSG is frequently associated with obesity.

2. A renal biopsy is not mandatory in this patient. It is also somewhat risky in view of previous nephrectomy.

3. Whether the patient has diabetic nephropathy or FSG, treatment is aimed at preventing further nephron loss. Systemic blood pressure should be controlled (diastolic pressure<85 mm Hg). Moderate protein "restriction" (0.6 to 0.8 g/kg/day) and ACE inhibitor (captopril, enalapril) therapy may lower intraglomerular hydrostatic pressure and slow progressive nephron loss. Blood sugar should be controlled at a reasonable level although its relationship to stabilization of renal function is less clear.

No specific therapy is available for either diabetic nephropathy or FSG. In addition, patients with only one kidney should undergo an open renal biopsy (requiring general anesthesia). Nevertheless, although a renal biopsy was recommended but the patient refused.

Case 4-2: *Discussion*

1. This case represents nephrotic syndrome complicated by ARF—i.e., two distinct processes. The major diagnostic alternative to explain the nephrosis and acute azotemia would be RPGN. However, the clear antecedent history of normal renal function, 4 + proteinuria, and bland urinary sediment make RPGN unlikely.

In the diagnostic approach to nephrotic syndrome (see Fig. 4-4) one promptly considers fenoprofen as a potential cause. NSAIDs can produce nephrotic syndrome, usually with minimal changes by light microscopy. Other secondary causes (diabetic nephropathy, SLE, and amyloid/neoplasia) were reasonably excluded by history, normal sugars, and negative serologies. The C3 and C4 were normal. In adults, primary (idiopathic) glomerular disease is less likely but must be considered.

2. The development of ARF in a patient with nephrotic syndrome (as in any patient) could be caused by glomerular (progression to RPGN), interstitial (acute interstitial nephritis due to NSAIDs), vascular disease (acute renal vein thrombosis) or ATN. In this patient, one must suspect an adverse interaction between the NSAID (fenoprofen) and triamterene (Maxide). This combination can cause ARF in as many as 50% of individuals, with or without demonstrable acute interstitial nephritis.

3. In this case, both fenoprofen and Maxide were discontinued. The creatinine rose to 12 mg/dl and supportive dialysis was instituted. Administration of corticosteroids was initiated (1 mg/kg/day). After 12 days without improvement (and because her nephrologist was getting anxious) a renal biopsy was performed. It showed minimal-change GN (normal light, no immunoglobulins, and foot process fusion by electron microscopy) and one small focus of interstitial inflammation.

The biopsy was believed to be consistent with minimal-change GN due to fenoprofen and drug-induced (fenoprofen and triamterene) interstitial nephritis that resolved perhaps as a result of treatment with steriods. No changes were made in therapy. Over the next 3 weeks, all abnormalities completely resolved and renal function returned to normal.

Case 4-3: *Discussion*

1. This patient has RPGN characterized by proteinuria, hematuria, RBC casts, and a rapid deterioration of renal function over a period of weeks to months.

2. In the diagnostic approach to RPGN (see Fig. 4-6) one considers nephritic diseases, vasculitis, and Goodpasture's syndrome before assuming the condition is idiopathic (as is the case in 60% of patients). The finding of hypocomplementemia in this patient were a C3 of 64 (N = 84 to 140) and a C4 of 12 (N = 16 to 30). These findings makes a nephritic disease a more likely diagnosis (see Table 4-9). PSGN was excluded by a negative history, ASO, and ASK. MPGN (unless secondary to some underlying disease such as SLE or infection) would be very unusual in an 83-year-old patient. With her history of previous endocarditis and a prosthetic aortic valve, bacterial endocarditis should be diligently excluded by repeated blood cultures, examination, and echocardiography. The ANA was 1:5120 and anti-DNA was 1:20, establishing a diagnosis of SLE. Her seizure was believed to be caused by lupus cerebritis (not uremia). Her protime did not fully correct with vitamin K. Both PT and PTT failed to correct with a 1:1 mix with normal plasma, suggesting the presence of a lupus circulating anticoagulant.

3. Renal biopsy showed a diffuse proliferative GN with numerous cellular and fibrous crescents (in 10 of 14 glomeruli). Some glomeruli were completely sclerosed and hyalinized. Granular IgG and C3, and to lesser extent IgM and IgA were seen by fluorescence microscopy. The biopsy was consistent with SLE.

References

Alpers CE, Cotran RS. Neoplasia and glomerular injury. Kidney Int 1986; 30:465–473.

Austin HA, Klippel JH, Balow JE, et al. Therapy of lupus nephritis: controlled trial of prednisone and cytotoxic drugs. N Engl J Med 1986; 314:614–619.

Austin HA, Muenz LR, Joyce KM. Prognostic factors in lupus nephritis: contribution of renal histologic data. Am J Med 1983; 75:382–391.

Berger J. IgA glomerular deposits in renal disease. Transplant Proc 1969; 1:939–944.

Couser WG. Rapidly progressive glomerulonephritis: classification, pathogenetic mechanisms, and therapy. Am J Kidney Dis 1988; 11:449–464.

Felson DT, Anderson J. Evidence for the superiority of immunosuppressive drugs and prednisone over prednisone alone in lupus nephritis: results of a pooled analysis. N Engl J Med 1984; 311:1528–1533.

Grünfeld JP. The clinical spectrum of hereditary nephritis. Kidney Int 1985; 27:83–92.

McCune WJ, Golbus J, Zeldes W, et al. Clinical and immunologic effects of monthly administration of intravenous cyclophosphamide in severe systemic lupus erythematosus. N Engl J Med 1988; 318:1423–1431.

Mogensen CE, Christersen CK, Vigstrup J. Early microalbuminuria, glomerular hyperfiltration, and late nephropathy and proliferative retinopathy. Diabetic Neph 1986; 5:37–39.

Sinniah R. IgA mesangial nephropathy: Berger's disease. Am J Nephrol 1985; 5:73–83.

Tejani A, Nicastri AD. Mesangial IgM nephropathy. Nephron 1983; 35:1–5.

5 Interstitial Nephritis

- Case Presentations
- Acute Interstitial Nephritis
- Chronic Interstitial Nephritis
- Diagnostic Approach
- Case Discussions

Case 5-1

A 46-year-old man presented with azotemia (BUN of 42 mg/dl, creatinine of 2.5 mg/dl) that was discovered during a recent hospitalization for a bleeding duodenal ulcer. He was asymptomatic, had had no previous kidney infections, stones, or urinary abnormality. Ten years earlier he was found to have hypertension and was administered hydrochlorothiazide, 50 mg daily, which he was still taking at the time of his presentation with azotemia. His past history was otherwise unremarkable. There was no history of chronic use of analgesics, chronic pain syndrome, or chronic arthritis, although he had occasional flare-ups of gout. Family history was negative for hypertension and renal disease. The patient did not smoke or drink alcohol. For 23 years he worked for a battery manufacturing company, where he continued to work at the time of presentation.

Blood pressure was 184/108 (supine and sitting). Fundi showed Grade II hypertensive retinopathy, and no gouty tophi were observed. The examination was otherwise negative. Urinanalysis showed a SG of 1.018 and trace protein of eight to ten WBC/hpf, four to six RBC/hpf. Urine culture was negative. The following table shows the results of laboratory tests.

Hgb	10.2 g/dl
Hct	32.5 %
WBC count	5,300
Platelet count	217,000
ESR	23.0 mm
Na	143.0 mEq/L
K	5.2 mEq/L
Cl	110.0 mEq/L
HCO_3	22.0 mEq/L
BUN	42.0 mg/dl
Creatinine	2.5 mg/dl
Ca	9.9 mg/dl
PO_4	3.4 mg/dl
Uric acid	8.3 mg/dl
Total protein	7.2 g/dl
Albumin	4.2 g/dl

Questions

1. What are the potential causes of his azotemia?
2. How might one confirm the diagnosis?

Case 5-2

A 43-year-old woman was admitted for weakness, generalized edema, proteinuria (4+) and renal insufficiency (BUN of 85 mg/dl, creatinine of 6.6 mg/dl).

Eight months earlier she had begun taking fenoprofen for joint pains. She was then asymptomatic for 7 months, at which point she suffered a severe "flu" characterized by sore throat, nausea, vomiting, headache, and extreme fatigue, all of which resolved over a

2-week period without specific therapy. However, 2 weeks before admission she began to have generalized edema, and her physician prescribed triamterene/hydrochlorothiazide (Maxide). Her blood pressure was 150/100, and she had a BUN of 27 mg/dl, a creatinine of 1.1 mg/dl, and a urine protein of 3+ at that time.

After admission to the hospital, physical examination showed the patient to be moderately obese and afebrile, with normal fundi, no adenopathy or rash, and a 2+ sacral edema and 3+ peripheral edema. The examination was otherwise normal. The following table shows the results of laboratory tests and urinalysis.

Laboratory		*Urinalysis*	
Hgb	10.2 g/dl	SG	1.024
Hct	31 %	Protein	4+
WBC count	11,600	Glucose	Negative
		RBC	4–6/hpf (without RBC casts)
Na	143.0 mEq/L	WBC	20–30/hpf
K	5.8 mEq/L		
Cl	114.0 mEq/L	24-hour urine	11.8 g protein
HCO₃	18.0 mEq/L	Urine culture	Negative
BUN	85.0 mg/dL		
Creatinine	6.6 mg/dl		
Ca	8.2 mg/dl		
PO₄	6.9 mg/dl		
Total protein	6.3 g/dl		
Albumin	3.1 g/dl		
Cholesterol	463 mg/dl		

Questions

What are the likely causes to explain the acute azotemia?

Case 5-3

A 54-year-old man was admitted for evaluation of gross hematuria and azotemia. He had no acute symptoms until he began passing grossly bloody urine 5 days earlier. There was no skin rash, change in his stool, respiratory symptoms, or arthralgia.

He had been disabled for several years because of a chronic low back syndrome with chronic pain. He adamantly denied having used analgesic preparations. He had no previous kidney problems but had taken blood pressure pills for 3 to 5 years. According to hospital records, 8 years earlier his BUN was 9 mg/dl and his creatinine was 1.2 mg/dl; 3 years earlier his BUN and creatinine were 23 mg/dl and 2.1 mg/dl, respectively. He had received recurrent phlebotomy for secondary erythrocytosis.

Physical examination revealed a blood pressure of 164/96. There was Grade I hypertensive retinopathy. The patient was moderately obese. No rash, edema, and pulmonary or neurologic abnormalities were found. Stool was heme negative.

Urinalysis revealed 1+ protein and 20 to 30 RBC/hpf. RBC surfaces were smooth and no dysmorphic changes were noted. There were ten to 20 WBC/hpf; urine culture was negative. Results of other pertinent laboratory tests are shown in the following table.

Hgb	11.4 g/dl
Hct	37.5 %
Platelet count	210,000
ESR	32 mm
Na	142 mEq/L
K	4.9 mEq/L
Cl	108 mEq/L
HCO_3	21 mEq/L
Glucose	114 mg/dl
BUN	39 mg/dl
Creatinine	4.2 mg/dl
Ca	8.5 mg/dl
PO_4	4.8 mg/dl
Uric Acid	6.1 mg/dl

Questions

1. What is the likely cause of his azotemia?
2. What are the most likely causes of his hematuria?

Case 5-4

A 44-year-old man was admitted for severe bilateral lower abdominal and epigastric pain (worse on the left side). The patient presented with significant azotemia (BUN of 34 g/dl, creatinine of 4.8 mg/dl). He was completely healthy until 2 days earlier, at which time the pain began. He had had no dysuria or hematuria. Nausea and vomiting occurred on the morning of admission. He had not moved his bowels for 48 hours.

His past medical history and family history were completely normal. He worked as a policeman, was taking no medication, and denied using alcohol or illegal drugs. There was no history of foreign travel. He was a suburban resident and had no pets or recent contact with animals.

Physical examination showed a blood pressure of 132/78, a pulse rate of 92 beats per minute, and a temperature of 37.4°C. There was no adenopathy, cardiac murmur, or rub. The lungs were clear. Abdominal examination showed diffuse abdominal tenderness without rebound. Bowel sounds were normal. There was marked bilateral flank tenderness. The remainder of the examination was normal.

Renal ultrasonography showed bilaterally enlarged kidneys without obstruction. The urinalysis revealed 1 + protein, 20 to 30 WBC/hpf, WBC casts, four to six RBC/hpf without RBC casts or dysmorphic cells. There was no bacteriuria. Urine culture was negative. Results of other pertinent laboratory tests are shown in the following table.

Hgb	13.9 g
WBC	13,800*
Na	140 mEq/L
K	3.8 mEq/L
Cl	105 mEq/L
HCO_3	23 mEq/L
BUN	34 mg/dl
Creatinine	4.8 mg/dl
Amylase	320
LDH	175

* 73 segs, 20 lymphs, 5 monos, 2 eos.

Over the next several days the patient developed bilateral testicular pain and swelling, dyspnea with a room air partial pressure of oxygen (PO_2) of 54, diffuse interstitial markings as demonstrated by chest radiographs, and intermittent confusion and headache. All cultures were negative. He received broad-spectrum antibiotics for 2 days. Renal function remained unchanged.

Questions

1. What is the most likely cause of his azotemia?
2. What diagnostic tests should be performed?

Interstitial nephritis refers to a heterogenous group of diseases that influence renal function primarily by affecting the renal tubules and interstitium. We use the term somewhat generically to include those disorders for which a direct renal tubular cell effect may be primary (tubulointerstitial nephritis) or for which the inflammatory component may be minimal (interstitial nephropathy).

Interstitial nephritis can be divided into two clinically distinct syndromes: *acute* and *chronic* interstitial nephritis. Both may share common clinical features, such as mild to moderate proteinuria, occasional hypertension, pyuria, and a variety of tubular function abnormalities (hyperkalemia, hyperchloremic acidosis, salt and water wasting). However, acute interstitial nephritis is usually a more fulminant condition, often presenting with flank pain, WBC casts, gross hematuria, and acute renal failure. Chronic interstitial nephritis is much more indolent, with a bland urinary sediment and very slowly progressive azotemia. The distinction is more than temporal, however, since the etiologies, renal histology, and pathogenetic mechanism responsible for each syndrome may differ substantially.

Histologically, interstitial cellular infiltrates predominate over vascular or glomerular changes. The infiltrates may variably include mononuclear cells, lymphocytes, plasma cells, eosinophils, and polymorphonuclear leukocytes. Atrophy or loss of tubular epithelial cells is common. Acutely, interstitial edema is common, probably accounting grossly for the normal to large size of some kidneys, whereas significant fibrosis accounts for the smaller shrunken kidneys of chronic interstitial nephritis.

Acute Interstitial Nephritis

Although a variety of infectious, metabolic, and autoimmune diseases may cause acute interstitial nephritis (AIN) (Table 5-1), greater than 90% of cases are allergy-related and due to drug use. The most common clinical presentation is that of acute azotemia that is biochemically similar to acute tubular necrosis (see Table 3-10). However, the urine sediment distinguishes AIN with marked pyuria, WBC casts, eosinophiluria (when the AIN is al-

Table 5-1 Common Causes of Acute and Chronic Interstitial Nephritis

	Acute	*Chronic*
Drugs/Toxins	NSAIDs	Analgesics (APC)
	Penicillins	Lead
	Cephalosporins	Cyclosporine
	Sulfonamides	Nitrosureas
	Diuretics	Lithium
Infections	Bacteria	Pyelonephritis
	Viruses	Anatomic
		Vesico-ureteral reflex
		Stones
		Obstruction
		TB
Tubular toxicity/ obstruction	Uric acid	Gouty nephropathy
	Oxalate	Oxalate nephropathy
	Myeloma	Nephrocalcinosis
		Myeloma
Immune	SLE	SLE
	Sjögren's syndrome	Sjögren's syndrome
	Transplant rejection	Transplant rejection
Hereditary		Polycystic kidney
		Medullary cystic disease
		Medullary sponge kidney

lergy-related), and usually an absence of the coarse granular casts typical of ATN.

Causes

Drugs

Drug-induced allergic interstitial nephritis accounts for 90% of AIN and roughly 10% of all ARF. Various agents (Table 5-2) may produce the syndrome. Of these, antibiotics (penicillin, cephalosporins, sulfonamides) and nonsteroidal anti-inflammatory drugs predominate. The sulfonamide-derived diuretics (thiazides, furosemide, bumetanide, and metolazone) may also cause allergic AIN.

The time of onset is variable, usually days to weeks after the patient begins taking antibiotics, but as long as weeks to months after taking NSAIDs. Most cases of AIN are idiosyncratic and not dose-related. Patients may have fever, skin rash, or eosinophilia, although only 30% will have all three. Arthralgias are also common. Eosinophiluria, when tested by Hansel's stain, is present in most cases of antibiotic-related disease. Eosinophilia and eosinophiluria are less common with NSAID-related AIN. On renal biopsy, significant numbers of eosinophils are usually detected in the otherwise

Table 5-2 Drugs Known to Produce Allergy-Related Acute Interstitial Nephritis

Antibiotics	Diuretics
Penicillins	Furosemide
Cephalosporins	Bumetanide
Sulfonamides	Thiazides
Rifampin	Chlorthalidone
NSAIDs	Triamterene*
Fenoprofen	Miscellaneous
Indomethacin	Allopurinol
Mefenamic acid	Captopril
Naproxen	Cimetidine
Tolmetin	Phenytoin

*Apparent synergistic toxicity with NSAIDs.

nonspecific acute inflammatory infiltrates. The syndrome should resolve with discontinuation of the offending agent. Steroids may accelerate recovery.

The pathogenesis of drug-induced AIN is unknown. Antibodies against the tubular basement membrane are documented in patients with methicillin-induced nephritis, but immunoglobulins and complements are not demonstrated in most cases. In many cases, cellular infiltrates are T-lymphocytes, suggesting that cell-mediated delayed hypersensitivity may mediate the inflammation. In other cases of AIN such as systemic lupus erythematosus and Sjögren's syndrome, immune complexes are likely to be pathogenetic.

The simultaneous occurrence of nephrotic syndrome with allergy-related AIN is commonly seen in patients who use NSAIDs. Histologically, the glomeruli show minimal-change (Nil) disease, with foot process fusion by electron microscopy. This may be a secondary phenomenon caused by lymphokines released from activated T cells involved in the acute inflammatory response. Alternatively, abnormal immune response may make patients with pre-existing Nil disease more susceptible to AIN. Decreases in renal blood flow and GFR due to NSAIDs could also contribute to this syndrome.

Infections

Acute pyelonephritis is AIN caused by direct interstitial invasion of bacteria. Believed usually to ascend from the lower urinary tract, the bacteria may also be blood-borne. Fever, flank pain, and leukocytosis are common, and urinary culture should reveal the organism (whereas with chronic pyelonephritis, the urine culture is often negative). Although unusual, repeated bouts of acute pyelonephritis can lead to chronic renal failure. This is much more likely to occur with a coincident anatomic defect or obstruction (reflux, stone, neurogenic bladder), as described later in this chapter.

AIN may also arise indirectly as a result of systemic infection with other bacteria, mycoplasma, brucellosis, *Legionella,* leptospirosis, toxoplasmosis, leprosy, and certain viruses (mononucleosis, measles, and rarely, mumps). Viruses may be responsible for many of the cases labelled "idiopathic" AIN.

Tubular Toxicity

Patients may present clinically with AIN when the primary insult appears to involve obstruction or direct toxicity to the intrarenal tubules. *Tubular cell injury* and interstitial inflammation are thought to result secondarily to this intratubular obstruction. This is seen with crystals of uric acid, oxalate, and multiple myeloma.

Acute *uric acid nephropathy,* usually a cause of oliguric ARF, results from acute precipitation of uric acid in the renal tubules. It is primarily seen in patients with lymphoproliferative or myeloproliferative disease after treatment with chemotherapy. The serum uric acid concentration is usually greater than 18 mg/dl. Interstitial and tubular uric acid deposition is aggravated by hyperuricemia (and subsequent uricosuria), volume depletion, and acid urinary pH. Prevention by volume expansion, allopurinol, and urinary alkalinization (IV $NaHCO_3$ and/or acetazolamide) is most important. If ARF occurs, hemodialysis is extremely effective in removing uric acid, after which total recovery of renal function is expected promptly.

A similar syndrome can occur with intratubular oxalate deposition associated with acute ethylene glycol poisoning and methoxyflurane anesthesia. These acute forms of uric acid and oxalate nephropathy are quite distinct from their chronic counterparts.

Immune Disorders

Multiple myeloma and a variety of immune disorders may also present as AIN. More commonly, these diseases produce an indolent chronic interstitial nephritis, and as such, are discussed in the following section.

Chronic Interstitial Nephritis

Patients with chronic interstitial nephritis (CIN) are usually discovered during evaluation of asymptomatic azotemia. In addition to the usual features of interstitial disease, an anemia out of proportion to the decrease in the glomerular filtration rate is common.

Broad casts may be seen in the urine sediment. With progressive loss of renal function, there may also be clinical and histologic evidence of glomerular involvement. Therefore, with CIN, albuminuria is not unusual and renal biopsies often show focal and segmental glomerular scarring and periglomerular fibrosis. Interstitial fibrosis usually exceeds cellular infiltrates late in the course of CIN.

Like AIN, CIN is produced by a variety of insults categorized generally as drugs and toxins, infections, and tubular, hereditary, and immune disorders (see Table 5-1). Unlike AIN, the responsible etiologic agents and pathogenesis in each category may be quite different. In fact, with rare exceptions (e.g., rare cases of acute pyelonephritis, cyclosporine, transplant rejection), AIN does not progress to CIN.

Causes

Drugs and Toxins

Analgesics (aspirin, phenacetin, acetaminophen, and NSAIDs), heavy metals (lead, cadmium), and other drugs (cyclosporine, lithium, nitrosureas, platinum) predominate in this category. *Analgesic nephropathy* refers to the chronic interstitial inflammation and scarring caused by prolonged consumption of non-narcotic analgesic compounds. The syndrome can apparently result from the isolated use of aspirin, phenacetin, acetaminophen, and the newer NSAIDs. However, combinations of these agents (aspirin plus either phenacetin or its metabolite, acetaminophen) produce a synergistic toxicity and are responsible for most cases. Rough estimates are that at least 2 kg (cumulative dose) of this combination or 4 kg of aspirin or acetominophen alone are necessary to produce the syndrome. This translates to four to six tablets daily for 4 to 6 years for the combination products.

The synergistic toxicity of aspirin and phenacetin/acetaminophen appears to result from a combined toxic and hemodynamic effect. Aspirin-induced decreases in renal blood flow may aggravate a nephrotoxic effect of an acetaminophen metabolite. Because these agents are concentrated in the inner renal medulla (papilla), where renal blood flow is most compromised, it is not surprising that inflammation, fibrosis, and necrosis are first evident in this area of the kidney. The lesion progresses to involve the entire medulla and papilla, eventually resulting in papillary necrosis and secondary cortical scarring. Despite the progressive nature of chronic renal insufficiency in most diseases, current evidence suggests that if the analgesics are discontinued, the progression of analgesic nephropathy may be retarded or even reversed.

A major impediment to diagnosing analgesic nephropathy is obtaining a reliable history of analgesic consumption, a fact which may partially explain the wide geographic variation in incidence worldwide. The diagnosis should be suspected if the patient simultaneously has acid peptic disease, iron deficiency anemia, or a chronic pain syndrome such as headache, arthropathy, or other musculoskeletal disorder. Indeed, close questioning about the severity and therapy required to control the chronic pain will often yield a more accurate history. Questioning family members usually improves the history substantially.

CIN should be viewed as only one of several syndromes associated with aspirin/acetaminophen use (Table 5-3). Microhematuria and enzymuria (N-acetyl glucosaminidase, B_2 microglobin) likely reflect mild tubular injury. Defects in urinary concentration may occur as renal medullary blood flow is compromised. Renal papillary necrosis may occur without severe renal insufficiency. Gross hematuria, renal colic, and acute obstructive uropathy can result from sloughed necrotic papilla. Finally, there exists a strong association between chronic analgesic use and transitional cell carcinoma, particularly of the renal pelvis and ureters. The incidence of a simultaneous transitional cell carcinoma in patients with analgesic nephropathy is estimated to be 5 to 10%.

Chronic Lead Exposure

Lead nephropathy refers to CIN resulting from chronic exposure to lead, usually from industrial sources (lead-containing paint, battery manufacturing, lead-mining) or illegally distilled al-

**Table 5-3 Renal Syndromes Associated
with Aspirin**

Microhematuria

Enzymuria (NAG)

Salt and water retention

Urinary concentration defects

Functional decline in GFR

Chronic interstitial nephritis

Papillary necrosis
  Gross hematuria
  Obstruction
  Colic

Transitional cell carcinoma

cohol. In addition to renal insufficiency, proximal tubular dysfunction with aminoaciduria, glycosuria, and hyperchloremic acidosis is common. Uric acid excretion is decreased, however, often causing hyperuricemia and gout. Encephalopathy, hypochromic microcytic anemia, and peripheral neuropathy are also associated with lead toxicity.

Blood levels unfortunately do not detect chronic lead exposure or body-lead burden. Measurement of 24-hour urinary lead excretion (72-hour in patients with renal insufficiency) after intramuscular administration of EDTA is the only reliable index of severe chronic lead exposure. A 24- to 72-hour urinary lead excretion of greater than 600 µg is highly suggestive of lead nephropathy.

Lead nephropathy is an underdiagnosed condition. Hypertensive and gouty patients with azotemia have a significantly higher urinary lead excretion after EDTA than those without renal insufficiency, suggesting that lead may be etiologic in some patients designated as having hypertensive nephrosclerosis or gouty nephropathy. Indeed, the clinical triad of hypertension, hyperuricemia with gout, and chronic renal insufficiency should suggest lead nephropathy and encourage EDTA testing.

Infections

Bacteria are most commonly associated with this form of CIN. Chronic tuberculosis may also be responsible. *Regardless of etiology, it is generally accepted that a coincident anatomic abnormality of the urinary tract is necessary for most renal infections to progress to chronic renal insufficiency.*

Chronic pyelonephritis refers to CIN caused by recurrent or persistent bacterial infection. It is much less common than previously thought. The nonspecific clinical and histologic features of chronic pyelonephritis as well as a lack of appreciation of other forms of CIN (e.g., analgesic nephropathy, lead nephropathy) made this an overdiagnosed condition in the past. Nevertheless, chronic pyelonephritis remains an important and potentially preventable cause of CIN and end-stage renal disease.

Most renal parenchymal infections are believed to arise by the ascending route. With an otherwise normal urinary tract, these infections usually resolve and do not cause progressive intersititial inflammation. However, when urinary obstruction, stones, or *vesicoureteral reflux* (VUR) compromise urinary drainage, chronic parenchymal infection, inflammation, and fibrosis occur, even in the absence of active renal infection. Contraction of the renal papillae results, producing small kidneys with cortical scars overlying dilated calyces, all typical (and necessary) diagnostic features of chronic pyelonephritis by IVP.

VUR is common. Thirty to fifty percent of children younger than 5 years of age with urinary tract infection will have documented reflux. Estimates are that 20 to 30% of all chronic renal failure in adolescents is caused by VUR. However, in most cases, intrarenal reflux (calyceal-tubular reflux) is also necessary to produce interstitial fibrosis and progressive renal scarring. VUR without intrarenal reflux and infection does occur, but in both instances is much less likely to produce renal scars. A strong association between VUR and focal segmental glomerulosclerosis also exists, perhaps contributing to the proteinuria, hypertension, and progression to ESRD in these patients.

Because VUR tends to resolve spontaneously over time, a nonsurgical approach is warranted in all but extreme cases. Chronic prophylactic antibiotic therapy is indicated to prevent renal scarring. Surgery for ureteral reimplantation is reserved for cases of severe (Stage IV) reflux with progressive renal scarring and/or recurrent symptomatic pyelonephritis.

Tubular Toxicity/Obstruction

Although mechanical obstruction of the renal tubules by uric acid, oxalate crystals or myeloma light-chains is probably the proximate cause of AIN, it appears to play a lesser role in the pathogenesis of CIN. Rather, interstitial crystalline or light-chain deposition is believed to be primarily responsible for the chronic interstitial inflammatory and fibrotic reaction.

Chronic urate (gouty) nephropathy results from medullary interstitial deposition of monosodium urate and subsequent giant cell reaction with interstitial fibrosis and tubular cell atrophy. It usually occurs in patients with long-standing hyperuricemia and tophaceous gout, although there is little evidence that hyperuricemia per se is deleterious to renal function. In most patients with urate nephropathy, uric acid lithiasis, pyelonephritis, hypertension, and/or glomerulosclerosis contribute substantially to chronic renal damage. The disease is slowly progressive and probably irreversible. Therefore, allopurinol therapy is not necessary except for treating concomitant gouty arthritis or uric acid stones. Uricosuric agents should be avoided.

A similar syndrome can arise from interstitial deposition of oxalate. Termed *chronic oxalate nephropathy,* it is usually caused by primary hyperoxaluria (a rare genetic amino acid transport disorder) or by large intestinal hyperabsorption of oxalate that occurs after small bowel resection, Crohn's disease, or intestinal bypass surgery. Nephrolithiasis, chronic pyelonephritis, and hypertension further compromise renal function.

Nephrocalcinosis is the interstitial deposition of calcium and phosphate crystals usually seen with chronic hypercalcemia and occasionally with isolated hypercalciuria. Calcium is also a tubular cell toxin such that obstructing casts of degenerating tubular cells are also common. This syndrome is aggravated not only by stones, but also by the nephrogenic diabetes insipidus, decreased glomerular permeability, and hemodynamic effects of hypercalcemia, regardless of etiology. Hyperparathyroidism, distal renal tubular acidosis, and sarcoidosis are commonly complicated by hypercalciuria and nephrocalcinosis.

Myeloma Kidney

Figure 5-1 shows the probable pathophysiology of *myeloma kidney.* Light-chains, freely filtered at the glomerulus, appear to be nephrotoxic to proximal tubular cells. Indeed, crystalline deposits of light-chains are identified in proximal epithelia. In addition, proteinaceous casts in distal renal tubules are regularly demonstrated by renal histology. These casts likely cause partial tubular obstruction and distal epithelial damage. Tubular atrophy and a reactive interstitial infiltrate result from tubular cell damage.

Not surprisingly, clinical disorders of proximal (Fanconi's syndrome) and distal (nephrogenic diabetes insipidus, distal renal tubular acidosis) function are frequently seen with myeloma kidney. Other renal syndromes associated with multiple myeloma are listed in Table 5-4. "Light-chain nephropathy" refers to the linear deposition of light-chains along the glomerular and tubular basement

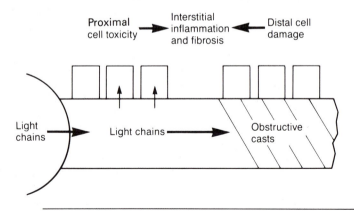

Figure 5-1: Schematic representation of the pathophysiology of myeloma kidney.

Table 5-4 Renal Syndromes Associated with Multiple Myeloma

Asymptomatic Bence Jones proteinuria
ARF
    Radiographic contrast
    Hypercalcemia
    Uric acid nephropathy
    Hyperviscosity

Glomerulonephritis
    Nephrotic syndrome (amyloid)
    Light-chain nephropathy

Interstitial nephritis (myeloma kidney)
    Fanconi's syndrome
    Nephrogenic diabetes insipidus
    Renal tubular acidosis

Nephrolithiasis

membranes occurring with or without the tubulointerstitial nephritis (myeloma kidney). Nephrotic syndrome caused by amyloid (AI) deposition is not uncommonly seen, particularly with long-standing myeloma. Chronic renal insufficiency will result in complications in 30 to 60% of patients with myeloma; 10% will develop ARF.

The clinician must remember that the presence of urinary light-chains does not necessarily mean that there will be multiple myeloma. Damage to the renal tubules and interstitium from any cause may prevent reabsorption of the physiologic quantities of light-chains normally filtered, resulting in "light-chain proteinuria." Immunoelectrophoresis distinguishes these polyclonal light-chains from the monoclonal proteins of myeloma. Monoclonal light-chains can also be demonstrated in the urine of patients with Waldenstöm's macroglobulinemia, as well as in 30% of patients with amyloidosis without myeloma and (rarely) those with B-cell lymphomas and leukemias.

Hereditary Diseases

Most hereditary diseases associated with interstitial nephritis are extremely rare (nail-patella, von Hippel Lindau disease, idiopathic multicentric osteolysis, Balkan nephritis). The renal cystic diseases are quite common, however, accounting for 10 to 15% of ESRD.

Autosomal dominant polycystic kidney disease (ADPKD) is the most dramatic of the cystic disorders. Both kidneys are enlarged with multiple cortical and medullary cysts of varying sizes. These cysts appear to be focal dilatations of nephrons, maintaining their functional capacity to transport sodium, potassium, hydrogen ions, and organic acids. Proximal and distal cysts are therefore readily distinguished by chemical analysis.

The renal tubular cysts are the most common of many structural anomalies in these patients. Cysts are commonly identified in the liver (30%), pancreas (15%), and (rarely) in the spleen. Diverticulosis is more frequent with ADPKD. The incidence of cardiac valvular abnormalities, especially mitral valve prolapse, is also increased. In addition, berry aneurysms of the cerebral vessels may result in complications in as many as 15% of all patients. Because the occurrence of berry aneurysms in ADPKD is familial, prospective cerebral angiograms should be considered for those patients with a family history of intracranial bleed or acute symptoms.

The spectrum of structural abnormalities seen in ADPKD has led some to speculate that a disorder of collagen is responsible for the renal cysts. Other theories propose that tubular obstruction caused by hyperplastic cells and/or disordered growth of tubular cells result in the cysts. Renal failure appears to result from compression of normal nephrons by cysts.

Patients usually present in the third and fourth decades of life with flank pain, urinary infection, or hematuria. Hypertension develops in 60 to 80% of these patients. Renal failure usually occurs by the age of 60 years, but relatively normal renal function may persist throughout life, despite kidneys grossly deformed by cysts. After years of dialysis, an acquired type of renal cystic disease may occur in patients with other causes of renal failure. Of concern is the propensity of ADPKD and especially of the acquired form of polycystic disease to malignant degeneration.

Patients with *medullary cystic disease* (MCD) usually present with severe renal failure between the ages of 30 and 40 years. Unless the patient has a severe salt-wasting syndrome, particularly common with MCD, he or she is usually asymptomatic. Autosomal recessive inheritance is documented in most, particularly those with the variant known as *juvenile nephronophthisis.* Autosomal dominant and sporadic cases are also documented.

Cysts are confined to the corticomedullary and medullary areas and appear to arise from distal tubules and collecting tubules. Secondary interstitial inflammation and fibrosis as well as glomerular sclerosis occur as the disease progresses invariably to uremia. Because of the relatively small size of the cysts, antemortem diagnosis is often difficult. The disease should be considered in young patients with severe azotemia and without history of urinary tract infection or reflux. There is no known treatment for this disease.

Medullary sponge kidney (MSK) is an anomaly frequently confused with MCD. This condition is characterized by ectasia of the papillary-collecting ducts with cavity formation and microcysts. Present in approximately one out of 5,000 normal persons, it is usually discovered as an incidental finding on IVP. Although 10 to 20% of these patients develop stones, urinary infection, or hematuria, the disorder does not progress to ESRD unless these complications are severe and/or obstruction occurs. Most cases are sporadic, but family tendencies are reported in approximately 10% of patients. Treatment is necessary only for complications.

The comparative features of ADPKD, MCD, and MSK are outlined in Table 5-5.

Diagnostic Approach

The basic diagnostic approach to patients with suspected interstitial nephritis is outlined in Figure 5-2. One must first entertain the possibility of interstitial nephritis. The characteristics of azotemia, hematuria, proteinuria, and pyuria suggestive of an interstitial process are outlined in Figure 5-3. Patients may present a broad range of clinical syndromes from an isolated asymptomatic abnormality to ARF to ESRD. Alternatively, interstitial nephritis may complicate the cause of underlying glomerular or renal vascular

Table 5-5 Comparative Features of Autosomal Dominant Polycystic Kidney Disease, Medullary Cystic Disease, and Medullary Sponge Kidney

	ADPKD	MCD	MSK
Inheritance	Autosomal dominant (90%) Sporadic (10%)	Autosomal recessive (70%) Autosomal dominant (15%) Sporadic (15%)	Familial in only 10 to 15%
Clinical features	Flank and abdominal pain Hematuria Hypertension Urinary infection	Usually asymptomatic until uremic Salt-wasting	Usually asymptomatic Stones Hematuria Urinary infection
ESRD incidence	80–90%	Near 100%	Rare
Patient age at onset of ESRD	30–60 yrs.	20–40 yrs.	
Location of cysts	Cortex and medulla	Medulla	Papilla

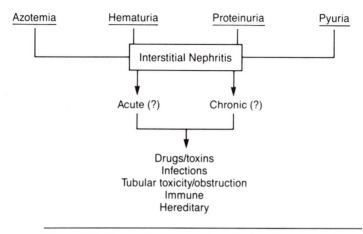

Figure 5-2: Diagnostic approach to patients with suspected interstitial nephritis. Details of these steps are outlined in Figures 5-3, 5-4, and Table 5-6.

disease. Whenever pyuria, WBC casts, minimal to mild proteinuria, and hyperkalemic hyperchloremic metabolic acidosis dominate the clinical presentation, interstitial nephritis should be considered.

Next, one must consider whether the interstitial process is acute or chronic. As in any other renal process, the history, rate of

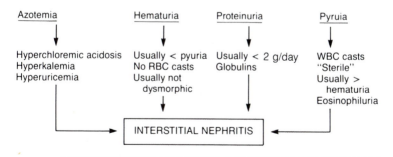

Figure 5-3: Diagnostic approach to interstitial nephritis (Step 1). Characteristics of azotemia, hematuria, proteinuria, and/or pyuria suggestive of interstitial nephritis are identified.

creatinine rise, serum albumin, hematocrit, and kidney size are important clues (Fig. 5-4).

Finally, the common diagnostic categories and specific etiologies of AIN or CIN can be considered (Tables 5-1 and 5-6). Most cases of AIN are drug- and allergy-related, making eosinophilia and eosinophiluria important diagnostic tests. A history and physical suggesting fever, chills, flank pain, tenderness, and dysuria is usually present with acute pyelonephritis. Radiographic studies to exclude anatomic (obstructive) lesions should be performed in these patients. The presence of uric acid or oxalate crystals in the urine would suggest that either of these are etiologic of AIN. Because the presentation of myeloma kidney is usually nonspecific, one must always maintain a high index of suspicion for this condition. Search for a paraprotein, bone marrow, and/or renal biopsy should confirm or exclude this possibility.

A renal biopsy is generally much less helpful with cases of CIN. Here, the clinical history is probably most important. *A carefully and objectively obtained history can virtually confirm or exclude the most common causes of CIN,* including analgesic nephropathy, lead toxicity, chronic pyelonephritis, gouty or oxalate nephropathy, immune disorders, and renal cystic disease.

Most cases of AIN are both treatable and reversible. CIN, on the other hand, is usually progressive and irreversible. Nevertheless, avoiding nephrotoxins (particularly in patients with analgesic ne-

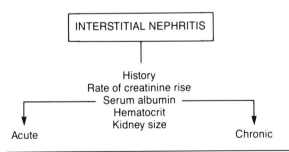

Figure 5-4: Diagnostic approach to interstitial nephritis (Step 2). Determining whether interstitial nephritis is acute or chronic.

Table 5-6 Diagnostic Approach to Interstitial Nephritis (Step 3): Diagnostic Categories and Specific Etiologies of Interstitial Nephritis are Considered*

	Acute			Chronic	
Etiology	Test	Treatment	Etiology	Test	Treatment
Drugs/toxins (allergy-related AIN)	Eosinophilia Eosinophiluria History/PE Renal Biopsy	Discontinue drug Steroids (?)	Drugs/toxins	History IVP EDTA	Discontinue offending agent
Infection	History/PE UA + Culture IVP/ultrasonography	Antibiotics	Infection	History IVP/ultrasonography Cultures TB skin test	Correct anatomy Antibiotics
Tubular obstruction	UA UPE SPE Bone marrow (?) Renal biopsy	Supportive Treatment of underlying condition	Tubular obstruction	History UPE SPE Bone marrow	Supportive Treatment of underlying condition
Immune	History ANA C3C4 Renal biopsy	Steroids ± immunosuppressives	Immune	History ANA C3C4	Steroid ± immunosuppressives
			Hereditary:	IVP/ultrasonography/CT Family history	Supportive

* See also Table 5-1.

PE = physical examination; UA = urinalysis; IVP = intravenous pyelography; UPE = urine protein electrophoresis; SPE = serum protein electrophoresis.

phropathy), correcting anatomic defects, and vigorously treating infections as well as providing nonspecific treatment for chronic renal insufficiency (low-protein diet, anti-hypertensives, ACE inhibitors) may effectively stabilize renal function in many patients with CIN.

Case 5-1: *Discussion*

1. The clinical findings of sterile pyuria, minimal proteinuria, relatively bland urinary sediment, and hyperchloremic metabolic acidosis with hyperkalemia out of proportion to the GFR suggest CIN.

Next, one should consider the causes and potential etiologies of CIN: drugs and toxins, infections, tubular toxicity/obstruction, and hereditary and immune diseases. There is no history of analgesic use or a chronic pain syndrome to suggest analgesic nephropathy. Lead toxicity is a possibility. Chronic pyelonephritis is unlikely since this patient does not have a history of stones or urinary infections; an IVP could exclude this possibility. Gouty nephropathy is possible in view of his history of gout, but this is usually seen with chronic tophaceous gout, which this patient does not have. Myeloma must certainly be considered an the urine checked for monoclonal proteins. Although the family history tends to exclude renal cystic diseases, renal sonography should be performed as well. Serologic markers should exclude autoimmune syndromes.

The clinical triad of renal insufficiency, hypertension, and gout, as well as the fact that this patient has a chronic exposure to industrial lead (battery manufacturing), strongly supports a diagnosis of lead nephropathy.

2. Lead nephropathy can be confirmed by demonstrating an excess in the 24- to 72-hour lead excretion after the intramuscular injection of the lead-chelating agent, calcium EDTA.

Case 5-2: *Discussion*

This patient presents features of both glomerular (11.8 g of proteinuria per day) and interstitial disease (hyperchloremic acidosis, sterile pyuria). One should therefore first strongly consider the diagnosis of vasculitis (see Chapter 6).

However, one must remember that NSAIDs can simultaneously

cause nephrotic syndrome (minimal-change histology) and AIN. This appears even more likely in this patient because he is taking fenoprofen, which is most commonly associated with this syndrome and triamterene, which produces a synergistic toxicity with nonsteroidal drugs.

Measurement of urinary eosinophils would be helpful diagnostically. A renal biopsy would probably not be necessary. The syndrome should resolve completely with discontinuation of the drugs and a brief course of corticosteroids.

Case 5-3: *Discussion*

1. This patient's chronic azotemia is likely caused by interstitial nephritis resulting in sterile pyuria, minimal proteinuria, and hyperchloremic acidosis.

The chronic low back syndrome and history of ulcer disease would suggest chronic use of analgesics. Although the patient denied this, a history obtained from his wife confirmed that the patient had been taking eight to ten aspirin and/or acetaminophen tablets daily for several years.

2. Although microscopic hematuria is common with interstitial nephritis, gross hematuria is unusual. Papillary necrosis could explain the gross hematuria and is strongly associated with analgesic nephropathy. Another possibility which must be excluded is transitional cell carcinoma, which occurs with greater frequency in long-term analgesic users.

Case 5-4: *Discussion*

1. The enlarged, swollen kidneys and WBC casts demonstrated in this patient virtually confirm an acute interstitial process. In the absence of drug ingestion or eosinophilia, "allergic" interstitial nephritis seems unlikely. One must therefore strongly suspect acute pyelonephritis.

There were no bacteria in any cultures of the blood and urine. Although the WBCs were elevated at 13,800, the differential was normal and the patient was without fever. One should strongly consider here a nonbacterial cause of pyelonephritis, particularly viruses.

The patient's other clinical manifestations indeed suggest inflammation in a variety of tissues; his clinical syndrome of meningitis, interstitial pneumonitis, pancreatitis, and orchitis is suggestive of adult mumps. Other infections to consider are cytomegalovirus, leptospirosis, and legionella.

2. IgM and IgG mumps antibody titration should be performed. In this patient, the IgM mumps antibody titer was elevated to greater than 1:10. In addition, his antimumps IgG titer rose from 1:160 during his acute illness to 1:640 during convalescence (25 days). This seems to confirm the clinical suspicion of AIN caused by mumps.

References

Batumen V, Landy E, Maesaka JK, Wedeen RP. Contribution of lead to hypertension with renal impairment. N Engl J Med 1983; 309:17–21.

Brown JH, McGeown MG. Reflux nephropathy as a cause of end stage renal failure. Clin Nephrol 1988; 29:103–104.

Eknoyan G. Analgesic nephrotoxicity and renal papillary necrosis. Semin Nephrol 1984; 4:65–76.

Gabow PA, Ikle DW, Holmes JH. Polycystic kidney disease: prospective analysis of nonazotemic patients and family members. Ann Intern Med 1984; 101:238–247.

Gonwa TA, Corbett VMD, Schey HM, Buckalew VM. Analgesic-associated nephropathy and transitional cell carcinoma of the urinary tract. Ann Intern Med 1980; 93:249–252.

Mujais SK, Quintanilla A. Chronic tubulo-interstitial nephritis: saga of the ubiquitous. Semin Nephrol 1988; 8:4–10.

Murray T, Goldberg M. Chronic interstitial nephritis: etiologic factors. Ann Intern Med 1975; 82:453–459.

Nolan CR, Anger MS, Kelleher SP. Eosinophiluria: a new method of detection and definition of the clinical spectrum. N Engl J Med 1986; 315:1516–1519.

Rota S, Mougenot B, Baudouin B, et al. Multiple myeloma and severe renal failure: a clinicopathologic study of outcome and prognosis in 34 patients. Medicine 1987; 66:126–137.

Wedeen RP. Occupational renal disease. Am J Kid Dis 1984; 3:241–257.

6 Vascular Disease of the Kidney

- Case Presentations

- Hypertensive Renal Vascular Disease

- Atherosclerotic Renal Vascular Diseases

- Systemic Vasculitic Syndromes That Affect the Kidney

- Microangiopathic Renal Vascular Disease

- Renal Vein Thrombosis

- Diagnostic Approach

- Case Discussions

Case 6-1

A 75-year-old man was admitted to the hospital for recurrent transient cerebral ischemic attacks. Past history revealed that the patient had chronic hypertension, had undergone an abdominal aortic aneurysmectomy 14 years earlier, and had chronic, stable renal insufficiency (BUN of 27 mg/dl, serum creatinine of 1.7 mg/dl). Physical examination showed a blood pressure of 132/78, and bilateral carotid and femoral bruits were present. Cataracts precluded funduscopic examination. The skin was normal.

The patient was systemically anticoagulated with heparin and underwent carotid angiography via the femoral approach. Severe occlusive carotid atherosclerosis was demonstrated.

After angiography, the patient complained of severe abdominal pain and distention. In addition, renal function deteriorated (creatinine of 6 mg/dl) despite good daily urine volume and stable blood pressure. Mild gastrointestinal bleeding necessitated discontinuation of heparin. New onset of atrial fibrillation with rapid ventricular response was controlled with digitalis.

Without specific therapy, the serum creatinine decreased to 3 mg/dl over 4 days. However, the serum creatinine increased to 12 mg/dl over the next week, and dialysis was initiated. Coincident with the rise in creatinine were oliguria, eosinophilia (8 to 16%) without eosinophiluria, hypocomplementemia (C3 and C4), a net-like erythematous rash of the lower extremities, and continued slow gastrointestinal bleeding. Upper endoscopy revealed stress ulcerations, and colonoscopy revealed colonic ulcerations consistent with ischemic colitis.

Questions

1. What is the most likely cause of the patient's chronic azotemia?
2. What is the cause of his acute transient and reversible renal deterioration after angiography?
3. What is the cause of his second, more severe renal deterioration?
4. What should be done to confirm the diagnosis?

Case 6-2

A 74-year-old man was hospitalized for hypertension and renal failure. He had stable, well-controlled hypertension for 15 years and mild azotemia (serum creatinine of 2 mg/dl). During the preceding 4 to 6 months, however, his blood pressure had become refractory to medical therapy. Two weeks earlier, captopril was added to his antihypertensive regimen of furosemide, hydralazine hydrochloride, nifedipine, and clonidine hydrochloride.

On admission, his blood pressure was 186/104. BUN and serum

creatinine were 86 mg/dl and 7.2 mg/dl, respectively. Examination showed Grade II fundi, as well as right carotid and abdominal and femoral bruits. Urinalysis showed 2+ proteinuria (quantitated at 800 mg/24 hr), but was otherwise normal. Renal nuclear scanning showed markedly reduced perfusion bilaterally. Renal ultrasonography showed no hydronephrosis, and the kidneys were 10 to 11 cm in length.

Captopril was discontinued and blood pressure was controlled with minoxidil. The renal function gradually returned to baseline without dialysis.

Questions

1. What is the most likely cause of the patient's chronic azotemia?
2. What is the most likely cause of the acute exacerbation of renal function?
3. Which patients are susceptible to this complication?
4. What further diagnostic tests should be considered?
5. What therapy should be considered?

Case 6-3

A 63-year-old woman was admitted to the hospital for fever, dyspnea, and renal insufficiency.

Seven months before admission, she began to have bilateral ear pain. A specialist diagnosed bilateral otitis media and treated her with antibiotics, which failed to resolve the problem. Although bilateral tubes were placed in the tympanic membranes, no improvement was noted. Eventually, treatment with corticosteroids was initiated, resulting in good resolution of the patient's symptoms. As her corticosteroid therapy was tapered and discontinued, the patient began to have significant chest congestion and cough. After failure with several different antibiotic courses, the patient was admitted to the hospital for further evaluation.

Two months earlier, conjunctivitis had been demonstrated on biopsy. Histology revealed nonspecific conjunctivitis.

Her physical examination showed a blood pressure of 146/80. She had tubes draining both middle ears. Eye examination was normal.

There was no tenderness over her sinuses. Chest examination revealed bibasilar rales with expiratory wheezes. She had a trace of peripheral edema, but no rash. Her WBC count was 23,000 with a normal differential and three eosinophils. Her sedimentation rate was 92. Urinalysis showed 2+ protein, 20 WBC/hpf, 6 RBC/hpf, and WBC and RBC casts. Her BUN was 47 mg/dl, and her creatinine was 2.4 mg/dl. Rheumatoid factor was positive at 1:640, ANA was 1:80, and C3 and C4 were normal. Chest x-ray examination revealed bilateral infiltrates. Sinus radiographs showed thickening of the mucous membranes. A bronchial biopsy showed subacute bronchitis, and biopsy of the sinuses showed acute and chronic sinusitis.

Questions

1. What is the cause of the patient's renal disease?
2. What other diagnoses are likely?
3. What would a renal biopsy show?
4. What treatment should be instituted?

Diseases primarily affecting renal vessels may interrupt perfusion to all nephrons, significantly influencing their function. Not surprisingly, the clinical features of these vascular diseases may therefore simultaneously mimic either a glomerular or interstitial process (see Table 2-3 and 6-1). Because of these variable and nonspecific findings, renal vascular diseases are often missed (e.g., renal thromboembolism), misdiagnosed (e.g., cholesterol renal emboli) or underappreciated (e.g., chronic atherosclerotic renal vascular disease). The clinician should always maintain a high index of suspicion for these renal vascular disorders.

Typically, primary vascular diseases of the kidney have non-nephrotic–range proteinuria. Both albumin and globulin are evident by electrophoresis. Hematuria and pyuria may both be present. Dysmorphic RBCs, RBC casts, and WBC casts with significant proteinuria that mimic the acute glomerulonephritic syndrome are often seen with renal vasculitis. More indolent vascular processes (e.g., hypertensive nephroscleroses) may appear as chronic interstitial nephritis. Thus, the simultaneous occurrence of features seem-

Table 6-1 Clinical Features Suggesting a Primary Renal Vascular Disease

Clinical Features	Comment
Hematuria	Microscopic or gross May have dysmorphic RBCs and/or RBC casts
Proteinuria	Variable quantity; usually < 2 g of protein/24 hrs Both albumin and globulins
Pyuria	Sterile WBC casts with acute vasculitis Eosinophils, occasionally with vasculitis or cholesterol emboli
Hypertension	Common—usually seen with azotemia
Small kidney size	Smooth cortical surface with small vessel disease; asymmetric with irregular surface with atherosclerotic disease

ingly typical of glomerular and interstitial disease should suggest a primary vascular process. *If the intern says glomerulonephritis and the resident says interstitial nephritis, think vascular disease.*

We arbitrarily divide vascular disease of the kidney into five diagnostic categories (Table 6-2): (1) hypertensive, (2) atherosclerotic, (3) vasculitic, (4) microangiopathic, and (5) venous.

Hypertensive Renal Vascular Disease

Hypertension is often identified as a proximate cause of chronic renal insufficiency and end-stage renal disease. Indeed, long-standing hypertension can cause intimal thickening and fibrosis of renal arteries as well as arterioles (arteriosclerosis). Subsequent ischemic damage to the renal parenchyma often produces shrunken, sclerotic glomeruli, tubular atrophy, dilatation, and interstitial fibrosis (nephrosclerosis). The resultant renal functional

Table 6-2 Renal Vascular Diseases

Hypertensive renal vascular disease
  Hypertensive nephrosclerosis
  Accelerated/malignant hypertension
	Microangiopathic
	  Hemolytic uremic syndromes
	  Progressive systemic sclerosis
	  Sickle cell nephropathy
	  Radiation nephritis
	  Preeclampsia

Atherosclerotic renal vascular disease
  Arterial/arteriolar sclerosis
  Thromboembolic
  Atheroembolic (cholesterol emboli)
	Renal vein thrombosis

Systemic vasculitis
  Polyarteritis nodosa
  Wegener's granulomatosis
  Hypersensitivity vasculitis
  Cryoglobulinemia
  Henoch-Schönlein purpura	

impairment is usually asymptomatic until the patient is uremic. The urine sediment is usually bland; urinary protein excretion is usually less than 1 g daily. Small kidneys without cortical scarring are typical. Cardiomegaly, left ventricular hypertrophy, and hypertensive retinopathy commonly accompany this disease. This clinical and histologic spectrum of chronic renal insufficiency caused by long-standing hypertension is termed *hypertensive renal vascular disease* (HRVD).

It is often difficult, and sometimes impossible, to distinguish HRVD from other causes of chronic azotemia. This is particularly true because hypertension so frequently accompanies and accelerates many diseases (e.g., analgesic nephropathy, lead nephropathy, chronic pyelonephritis, and chronic GN). HRVD is therefore diagnosed largely through exclusion and has no specific histologic or clinical features.

Hypertension may also cause acute renal failure or acutely aggravate any pre-existing renal parenchymal disease. Malignant hypertension produces prominent fibrinoid necrosis in small preglomerular arterioles, resulting acutely in an ischemic glomerulopathy. Glomerular shrinkage with basement membrane "wrinkling," fibrin microthrombi, and occasional crescents are seen. Microscopic hematuria, proteinuria, and often RBC casts are also seen, thus mimicking an acute GN. Anti-hypertensive therapy will usually

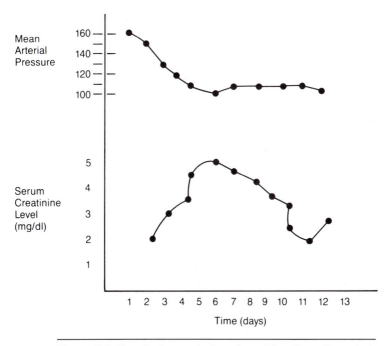

Figure 6-1: Transient exacerbation of renal function with control of malignant hypertension.

improve both the histologic and clinical picture of malignant hypertension, although transient worsening of renal function over a period of days to weeks is not uncommon (Fig. 6-1). If the serum creatinine is more than 5 to 6 mg/dl at the time of presentation, recovery of renal function cannot always be anticipated.

Atherosclerotic Renal Vascular Diseases

Atherosclerosis may affect renal function in several ways—for example, through renovascular hypertension (see Chapter 2), renal artery thromboembolism, diffuse cholesterol emboli, and *arteriosclerotic renal vascular disease* (ASRVD).

ASRVD refers to chronic renal insufficiency, presumably resulting from the indolent, progressive occlusion of small and large renal arteries caused by arteriosclerosis. Although one usually thinks of renovascular hypertension as resulting from renal atherosclerosis, chronic azotemia with or without hypertension is probably a more common result. ASRVD is analogous to the chronic ischemic organic brain syndrome or ischemic cardiomyopathy caused by progressive cerebral and coronary artery disease, respectively.

ASRVD should be considered in patients who have clinical features of renal vascular disease and evidence of generalized atherosclerosis. Vascular bruits are often present, and a history of previous stroke, myocardial infarction, or claudication is common. In fact, in one study, major renal artery occlusive disease is found in 25% of patients undergoing coronary angiography. Renal artery atherosclerosis has been documented in two-thirds of coronary patients who also have hypertension and azotemia. In addition, histologic studies confirm the usual presence of renal microvascular disease in patients with chronic atherosclerotic lesions of the renal arteries demonstrated angiographically.

The presence of renal atherosclerosis in a patient with chronic azotemia does not necessarily prove its causative role. Nevertheless, chronic azotemia can result from renal arteriosclerosis and in some cases can be reversed by revascularization. In addition, this disease will progress in 40 to 60% of patients over a period of months to years. In most cases, such progression correlates with a decrease in renal size and an increase in serum creatinine independent of blood pressure control.

Patients at high risk for disease progression can be considered for revascularization to preserve renal function, even in cases where there is no hypertension (Table 6-3). Therefore, those with mild to moderate azotemia that is believed to be secondary to ASRVD (other causes excluded) and with greater than 75% occlusion of one or both renal arteries might benefit from surgery or balloon angioplasty. If, however, the kidneys are small (<8 to 9 cm), the azotemia severe (creatinine>4 mg/dl), or a very delayed nephrogram is evident by arteriography, microvascular disease has likely progressed to an irreversible stage and revascularization is less likely to help.

Table 6-3 Patients with Atherosclerotic Renal Vascular Disease Who Might Be Candidates for Surgery to Preserve Renal Function

Those with serum creatinine level of 2–4 mg/dl (other causes excluded)

Those with greater than 75% occlusion as demonstrated by arteriography

Those with renal length greater than 9 cm

Prompt nephrogram on contrast study

Renal artery embolism (either thromboembolism or atheroembolism) is a frequently missed diagnosis. It should be considered whenever unexplained azotemia occurs in a patient with underlying atherosclerotic cardiac disease and arrhythmia. Thromboemboli are often of sufficient size to cause renal infarction. The acute onset of fever, flank and/or abdominal pain with nausea and vomiting are common (Table 6-4). Most patients will have an elevated serum lactate dehydrogenase with serum glutamic-oxaloacetic transaminase (SGOT), serum glutamic-pyruvic transaminase (SGPT), and serum alkaline phosphatase less likely to be increased. Acute

Table 6-4 Signs and Symptoms of Renal Artery Thromboembolism Causing Renal Infarction

Signs	Percentage of Patients
Acute azotemia	>90%
Increased LDH	>90%
Leukocytosis	>90%
Urinalysis	
Microhematuria	80%
Proteinuria ≥ 2+	70%
Sterile pyuria	70%
Fever	70%
Nausea, vomiting	50%
Abdominal pain	40%
Flank pain	40%

azotemia and leukocytosis are also very common. This constellation of findings may mimic those of an acute surgical abdomen, making the correct diagnosis very important.

Once suspected, the diagnosis can be confirmed by renal flow scan or arteriography. Without treatment, the symptoms will usually improve or resolve within days or weeks. Systemic anticoagulation may be necessary to improve renal function, and its use is suggested in most cases.

Atheroembolic renal artery disease (*cholesterol embolization*) may be more subtle and difficult to diagnose. This azotemic syndrome results from the occlusion of small arteries and arterioles by atheromatous material arising from ulcerated atherosclerotic plaques in the proximal circulation. The clinical manifestations are numerous and include ischemic changes of the lower extremities, such as livedo reticularis (red-blue mottling of the skin in a netlike appearance), painful muscles, mononeuropathies, and overt gangrene (Table 6-5). Pancreatitis and ischemic bowel with gastrointestinal bleeding are also common. Patients are usually oliguric with microhematuria, proteinuria, and sterile pyuria. Eosinophilia and eosinophiluria are common. Hypocomplementemia is also well documented. Because hypocomplementemia and the multisystem illness described above may mimic systemic vasculitis, cholesterol microemboli must always be considered in the differential diagnosis of vasculitis in elderly patients.

Table 6-5 Signs of Atheroembolic Renal Vascular Disease (Cholesterol Embolization)

Livedo reticularis

Myopathy

Mononeuropathy

Ischemic bowel

Pancreatitis

Microhematuria/proteinuria/sterile pyuria

Eosinophilia/eosinophiluria

Hypocomplementemia

Atheroembolic renal artery disease is usually seen in elderly patients with severe erosive disease of the aorta after an intravascular procedure (surgery or catheterization). Other cases may develop spontaneously or occur after systemic anticoagulation, presumably because the lysis of thrombus exposes an ulcerated plaque. The syndrome is documented by the microscopic finding of crystalline cholesterol deposits, usually identified by their typical biconvex, needle-shaped clefts on tissue biopsy (skin, bowel, kidney).

There is no known treatment for this syndrome. Nonspecific therapy aimed at the microcirculation (prazosin or calcium blockers) may be helpful. Spontaneous recovery does occur, particularly if a precipitating factor such as surgery or catheterization has already taken place. Anticoagulants should be avoided.

Systemic Vasculitic Syndromes That Affect the Kidney

Several of the systemic vasculitic syndromes may involve the renal circulation, resulting in a variable and nonspecific clinical picture. With these syndromes, there is no renal or glomerular lesion that is pathognomonic of vasculitis. At presentation, patients may have the nephrotic syndrome, rapidly progressive glomerulonephritis, or an asymptomatic renal abnormality. Fever, weight loss, anemia, leukocytosis, eosinophilia, and an elevated sedimentation rate may also be present. Despite these nonspecific features, systemic vasculitic diseases that affect the kidney can be divided into distinct clinical syndromes based upon their clinical and laboratory features (Table 6-6).

Polyasteritis Nodosa

Sixty to eighty percent of patients with *polyarteritis nodosa* (PAN) will have renal involvement. A necrotizing vasculitis and focal, segmental necrotizing GN may be seen, but often the renal biopsy will not demonstrate the vascular lesion. Immunofluorescence and electron microscopy usually show no changes other than a

Table 6-6 Clinical and Laboratory Features of Systemic Vasculitic Syndromes Affecting the Kidney

Syndrome	Vessel Involved	Renal Biopsy		
		LM	IF	EM
Polyarteritis nodosa	Small, medium muscular arteries	Focal segmental necrosis, crescents, collapse of capillaries, occasional microaneurysms	Neg	Neg
Wegener's granulomatosis	Aterioles	Focal segmental necrosis, crescents, collapse of capillaries, occasional microaneurysms Granulomata may be seen	Neg	Neg
Hypersensitivity vasculitis*	Arterioles, venules	Necrotizing vasculitis Lesions of similar age	Neg	Neg
Cryoglobulinemia	Arterioles, venules	Mesangial proliferative, intracapillary thrombosis	IgG IgM C3	Subendothelial deposits
Henoch-Schönlein purpura	Arterioles, venules	Occasional mesangial proliferative crescents	Mesangial IgA	Mesangial deposits

*Leukocytoclastic vasculitis, microscopic PAN, allergic vasculitis.
†Decreased with serum sickness. Varies with underlying disease. LM = light microscopy;

collapse and wrinkling of the glomerular basement membrane, which suggest ischemia as the cause of the glomerular lesion.

Multiple organs may be affected by PAN (see Table 6-6). Skin and lung are characteristically not involved, although asthma and eosinophilia may occur in the Churg-Strauss variant. The etiology is rarely determined, but as many as 30% of patients with PAN will have hepatitis B surface antigenemia, suggesting its pathogenic role in some patients.

Rapid evaluation is essential, since survival can be significantly improved with corticosteroid and cyclophosphamide therapy. Cytotoxic therapy should be withheld unless necrotizing vasculitis is

Table 6-6 (Continued)

C3	HB$_x$Ag (%)	Extrarenal Features	Treatment	Survival (Percentage of Patients Untreated/ Treated)
N	30%	GI bleeding/infarction Myositis/myalgia Arthralgia Mononeuropathy	Steroids, cytoxan	30%/70%
N	—	Sinusitis Pulmonary nodules/infiltrates Conjunctivitis Arthritis/Arthralgia Otitis	Steroids, cytoxan	20%/80%
N†	—	Skin purpura/petechial arthritis/arthralgia Neuropathy	Steroids ±	80%/80%
↓	10–20%	Pupura Arthritis/arthralgia Raynaud's disease	Pulse steroids, oral steroids, plasmapheresis	Varies
N	—	Arthritis, purpura, GI bleeding	Steroids ±	80%/80%

IF = immunofluorescence microscopy; N = normal; EM = electron microscopy; C3 = third component of complement.

demonstrated by biopsy of kidney, muscle, or nerve, or unless microaneurysms are identified by visceral arteriogram.

Wegener's Granulomatosis

Cyclophosphamide has also favorably influenced the survival of patients with *Wegener's granulomatosis.* In patients with this condition, renal biopsy shows a focal, segmental necrotizing GN similar to that of PAN, although granulomata are occasionally evident. However, granulomatous involvement of the nasopharynx, paranasal sinuses, and nodular cavitary pulmonary infiltrates clearly distinguish this syndrome from PAN. Conjunctivitis, iritis, otitis media, and involvement of joints, heart, skin, and nerves are also seen. The prognosis, however, is related to the degree of renal involvement at presentation.

Hypersensitivity Vasculitis

Hypersensitivity vasculitis (HSV) refers to a heterogenous group of diseases in which small vessel vasculitis usually develops 1 to 10 days after a single precipitating event, most commonly drug exposure. Generally, the lesions are at the same stage of development simultaneously—in contrast to the lesions of different stages so frequently encountered with PAN or Wegener's granulomatosis. Clinically, patients present with nephritic syndrome or asymptomatic hematuria. In addition to the kidney, the skin is typically affected with palpable purpura and/or petechiae, the most common manifestation.

HSV is occasionally seen in patients with a collagen vascular disease (systemic lupus erythematous, rheumatoid arthritis), lymphoreticular malignancy, or after administration of heterogenous protein (serum sickness). The disease is usually self-limited, and treatment with corticosteroids has little proven efficacy.

Cryoglobulinemia

Cryoglobulinemia refers to the presence of circulating immune complexes which precipitate in the cold and dissolve with rewarming. Cryoglobulins are classified into three types: (I) monoclonal immunoglobulins, such as the Bence Jones proteins; (II) monoclonal immunoglobulins (usually IgM) with activity against a polyclonal immunoglobulin (usually IgG); and (III) polyclonal immunoglobulins of one or more types. Cryoglobulins are not specific for any particular disease and, in fact, are encountered in a variety of conditions, including connective tissue diseases (SLE, Sjögren's syndrome, rheumatoid arthritis), infections (syphilis, subacute bacterial endocarditis, HB_sAg, cytomegalovirus, and others) and malignancies (chronic lymphocytic leukemia, lymphoma, myeloma). An idiopathic form, not associated with any underlying disease, is called *essential mixed cryoglobulinemia* (Type II).

A mesangioproliferative GN with positive immunofluorescence and subendothelial deposits by electron microscopy is usually responsible for the microhematuria, proteinuria, or nephritic syndrome commonly seen in these patients. Hypocomplementemia is common. Extrarenal manifestations include a purpuric/petechial rash, arthritis, mononeuropathy, Raynaud's phenomenon, and weakness. The clinical course is usually indolent and varies tremendously with the underlying disease. "Pulse" steroids and plasmapheresis appear effective for acute exacerbation.

Henoch-Schönlein

Henoch-Schönlein purpura (HSP) is the clinical tetrad of nephropathy (usually nephritic, occasionally RPGN), dermopathy (purpuric rash), arthropathy (arthritis or arthralgia) and gastroenteropathy (pain, bleeding, intussusception) caused by small-vessel IgA vasculitis. It is likely at the opposite end from Berger's (IgA) nephropathy in a spectrum of IgA-mediated immune complex diseases. The syndrome usually follows an acute viral infection or is perhaps the result of a food allergy. Although often transient and self-limited, the condition does recur. The prognosis is related to the severity of the clinical features, with 10 to 20% of cases progressing to ESRD. Corticosteroids have no proven efficacy but are often used to control the arthritis, rash, and occasional pleuropulmonary involvement.

Microangiopathic Renal Vascular Disease
Hemolytic Uremic Syndrome

Although diverse in origin and pathogenesis, the microangiopathic renal vascular diseases have in common primary vascular endothelial damage with subsequent localized intravascular coagulation.

The hemolytic uremic syndrome (HUS) refers to the clinical triad of ARF, thrombocytopenia, and microangiopathic hemolytic anemia. Actually, a host of diseases can produce similar features and can likewise be considered hemolytic uremic syndromes (Table 6-7). The idiopathic form is recognized most commonly in children and only occasionally in adults. It often develops after a viral-like syndrome or bacterial infection (shigellosis, *Salmonella, Escherichia coli, Pseudomonas*). Infection may also play a role in those cases associated with catastrophies of pregnancy such as septic abortion, abruptio placentae, or retained placenta. Alternatively, the syndrome may follow pregnancy by days to weeks and has been reported with estrogen-containing oral contraceptives, suggesting that hormones may be responsible for certain cases. Other drugs, particularly cancer chemotherapeutic agents, have been implicated. Finally, a hereditary or familial variety prone to recurrences also exists.

The differences between *thrombotic thrombocytopenic purpura* (TTP) and HUS seem to be more imagined than real. TTP generally occurs in older patients and presents with predominant neurologic manifestations and less severe renal involvement. Other organs such as the skin, liver, heart, muscle, and pancreas are also variably

Table 6-7 Hemolytic Uremic Syndromes

Idiopathic/postinfectious HUS
  Childhood
  Adult

Pregnancy-related HUS
  (Causes: septic abortion, abruptio placentae, retained placenta)

Postpartum HUS

Drug-induced HUS
  (Causes: oral contraceptives, mitomycin, cisplatin, bleomycin, Vinca alkaloid)

Malignancy HUS

Hereditary/familial HUS

Thrombotic thrombocytopenic purpura

involved in these syndromes. The syndromes thus appear to differ more in the extent and distribution of the thrombotic microangiopathy than in pathogenesis.

Histologically, intravascular coagulation with subintimal fibrin deposition and fibrin microthrombi is evident in arterioles. Subendothelial fibrin and fibrinoid necrosis are also present in glomeruli, appearing as electron-dense material on electron microscopy and "lighting up" with antifibrin immunofluorescence staining. Endothelial cell swelling and luminal narrowing result.

The prognosis varies depending on the age of the patient, the underlying cause of disease, and the degree of renal and central nervous system (CNS) involvement. Untreated, the idiopathic childhood variety is associated with an 80 to 90% survival rate. All other forms have a worse prognosis. Recurrent episodes are well documented, and recurrence is common in renal transplants. Uncontrolled trials using exchange transfusion, plasma infusion, or plasmapheresis appear to influence survival favorably.

Scleroderma

Obliterative vascular lesions also appear to be responsible for the renal manifestations of *progressive systemic sclerosis* (PSS) (scleroderma). In this condition, collagen accumulation in interlobular arteries and afferent arterioles ("onion-skinning") causes progressive narrowing of the vascular lumen and microinfarcts of glomeruli and interstitium. The glomerular changes resemble those of polyarteritis (i.e., an ischemic glomerulopathy). The interstitial changes vary from acute edema and tubular necrosis to chronic fibrosis and tubular atrophy, depending on the acuity and extent of the vascular lesion.

The clinical renal manifestations of PSS mirror this variable histologic picture. Thus, a spectrum of renal involvement exists, ranging from asymptomatic proteinuria (which may slowly progress to chronic renal insufficiency even without hypertension) to fulminant ARF and malignant hypertension. Indeed, the severity of hypertension appears to be the most reliable predictor of severe renal involvement and poor prognosis.

Sickle Cell Nephropathy

In patients who are homozygous for sickle hemoglobin, progressive occlusion of inner medullary arterioles (vasa recta circulation) can occur as the RBCs are exposed to dramatic changes in pH and tonicity. The resultant ischemia is likely responsible for the hematuria, renal infarction, patchy interstitial fibrosis, and papillary necrosis known as *sickle cell nephropathy*. A concentrating defect, acidification defect, hyperkalemia, and hyperuricemia are common functional changes. Patients who are heterozygous for the sickle cell gene may have similar abnormalities, although less frequent and severe.

Renal Vein Thrombosis

Although *renal vein thrombosis* (RVT) can occur in any hypercoagulable state (pregnancy, oral contraceptive-induced hormonal changes, cancer), it most typically complicates a pre-existing nephrotic syndrome, usually due to membranous or membranoproliferative GN. In such patients, an abrupt increase in urinary protein and an abrupt decrease in glomerular filtration rate or pulmonary embolism should prompt consideration of RVT.

Acute RVT may mimic renal thromboembolism with flank pain, fever, chills, hematuria, and elevated serum LDH. Enlargement of the involved kidney may be noted on intravenous pyelography, CT, or renal ultrasonography.

Alternatively, RVT may be more indolent or chronic and present with a constellation of findings, including variable proteinuria, hyperchloremic acidosis, hematuria, sterile pyuria, and inappropriate glucosuria. Patients may also demonstrate various coagulation abnormalities, such as elevated fibrin degradation products and platelets and decreased levels of antithrombin III and clotting factors V, VIII, and IX. Owing to the nonspecific nature of these features, the clinician must have a high index of suspicion if RVT is to be diagnosed.

The diagnostic procedure of choice is renal venography. Performing anticoagulation initially with heparin and subsequently with sodium warfarin (Coumadin) (usually for 6 months) will aid in thrombolysis and favorably influence the clinical course. Because recurrences are known to occur, patients should continue to receive antiplatelet drugs if the nephrotic syndrome or hypercoagulable state persists.

Diagnostic Approach

Figure 6-2 outlines a diagnostic approach to patients with possible renal vascular disease. This approach involves three major steps.

First, the clinical features suggesting the possibility of a primary renal vascular process are considered. The clinician must also be aware that, more often than with GN or interstitial nephritis, a patient with renal vascular disease is likely to have a systemic disease. Thus, involvement of multiple organs (e.g., brain, heart, lungs, gastrointestinal tract, skin) is an excellent clinical clue. Nevertheless, the clinical features of renal vascular disease are often nonspecific and show considerable overlap with the features of glomerular and interstitial diseases (see Tables 2-3 and 6-1). Not surprisingly, these diseases are often missed or misdiagnosed. One must therefore maintain a high index of suspicion for the possibility of renal vascular disease.

Second, one must consider the diagnostic categories of renal vascular disease: hypertensive, atherosclerotic, systemic vasculitic, microangiopathic, or venous disease. Once again, there may be considerable overlap between syndromes. For example, features of hypertension and diffuse atherosclerosis are often seen in the same patient, and in fact, HRVD and ASRVD often coexist. In addition, the distinction between vasculitic and microangiopathic diseases is often cloudy. Therefore, although one diagnostic category may seem the most likely, other possibilities should always be kept in mind.

Finally, each etiology in a given diagnostic category should be considered and confirmed by appropriate testing. Of the hypertensive diseases, chronic nephrosclerosis (HRVD) is essentially diagnosed through exclusion. Because it is often confused with chronic

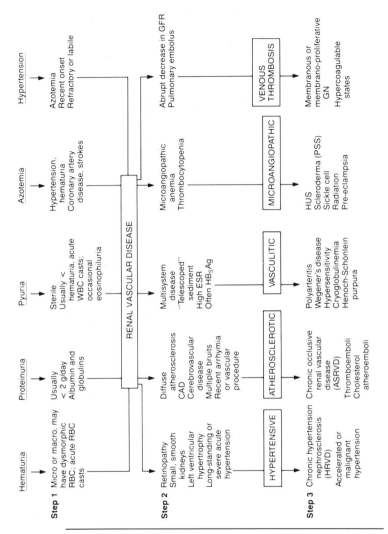

Figure 6-2: Diagnostic approach to the patient with renal vascular disease. Step 1: The clinical features suggesting the possibility of a primary renal vascular process are considered. Step 2: Clinical clues to a particular diagnostic category are considered. Considerable overlap exists. Step 3: The individual etiologies in each category are considered. CAD = coronary artery disease; ESR = erythrocyte sedimentation rate.

glomerular and particularly interstitial diseases, the diagnosis of HRVD is usually made after other renal vascular, glomerular, and interstitial diseases have been ruled out.

Accelerated or malignant hypertension is not easy to miss, but it may disguise an occult glomerulonephritic or vasculitic process. Atherosclerotic diseases are the most underappreciated, but are important to recognize because surgery or transluminal angioplasty may improve renal function in some patients (those with ASRVD). The clinical features differentiating the vasculitic diseases are displayed in Table 6-6. Although relatively rare and often missed, the vasculitic, microangiopathic, and veno-occlusive diseases are potentially fatal conditions that often respond to treatment, obligating the physician to be particularly diligent in making the correct diagnosis.

Case 6-1: *Discussion*

1. In this patient, renal vascular disease is suggested by his diffuse atherosclerotic disease and chronic hypertension. Certainly, chronic GN and interstitial nephritis are possible, although they are less likely.

2. The acute exacerbation in renal function after arteriography could be ascribed to acute radiographic contrast agents. The nonoliguric and transient nature of the renal failure are certainly consistent with this diagnosis. Another possible cause might be acute allergic interstitial nephritis. The most typical potential causes of this syndrome would be use of antibiotics, nonsteroidal anti-inflammatory drugs, and diuretics.

3. There are several possibilities to explain the patient's more severe renal deterioration late in his clinical course. The acute onset of atrial fibrillation with rapid ventricular response commonly precipitates renal thromboembolism. Again, acute drug reactions must also be considered. The clinical course, however, is most consistent with the syndrome of cholesterol atheroemboli. Indeed, the eosinophilia, hypocomplementemia, and rash (livedo reticularis) are quite typical of this syndrome. In addition, the ischemic colitis would suggest atheroemboli to the bowel.

4. Confirmation of the cholesterol atheroemboli syndrome is obtained by the presence of typical cholesterol clefts on tissue biopsy of involved skin or organs (e.g., the kidney). Occasionally, it also can be documented clinically by the presence of Hollenhorst's plaques on funduscopic examination. In this particular patient, the cholesterol atheroemboli were documented on biopsy of the ulcerative lesions in the ischemic colon.

Case 6-2: *Discussion*

1. The presence of long-standing hypertension and diffuse atherosclerotic disease would suggest renal vascular disease as a primary cause of this patient's chronic azotemia.

2. In this patient, the acute exacerbation of renal function is most likely caused by captopril therapy. Although captopril may sometimes cause an allergic interstitial nephritis, this is not likely to be the case in this patient because of the absence of eosinophilia or active urine sediment; it is more likely that captopril has induced a functional, hemodynamically mediated ARF (see Chapter 3).

3. In a patient with two kidneys, this is highly suggestive of bilateral renal artery stenosis, and in a patient with a solitary or transplanted kidney, it is suggestive of unilateral stenosis. This hemodynamically mediated renal failure likely occurs in 20 to 40% of these patients and is much more likely to occur in those patients who are taking diuretics. As in this patient, the renal failure is usually reversible after a period of days to weeks. Renal biopsy in these cases of hemodynamically mediated ARF will not show acute tubular necrosis.

4. Once the patient's renal function has recovered, one must consider whether or not surgery or angioplasty would be of benefit, not only for control of hypertension but also to preserve renal function. Arteriography should be performed. In this patient, the arteriogram showed an 80% stenosis of the right renal artery and a 90% stenosis of the left renal artery, as well as bilateral iliac and femoral arteriosclerosis. Renal vein renin studies failed to lateralize renin production to either kidney.

5. The relative preservation of renal size, mild renal insufficiency (serum creatinine 2 mg/dl), and high-grade renal artery stenoses suggest that this patient is a good surgical candidate for renal revascularization.

He did undergo bilateral renal revascularization with excellent results. Six months after surgery, his blood pressure was 132/78 while he was administered only 10 mg of nifedipine every 8 hours and 12.5 mg of chlorthalidone daily. In addition, his BUN and serum creatinine improved to 22 mg/dl and 1.1 mg/dl, respectively.

Case 6-3: *Discussion*

1. The presence of both RBC and WBC casts demonstrated on urinalysis suggest the possibility of renal vascular disease. The low-grade proteinuria and azotemia are likewise consistent with this diagnosis. In fact, the urinalysis is typical of a "telescope urinary sediment," suggesting acute preglomerular vasculitis. The obvious presence of a multisystem disease as well as a markedly elevated sedimentation rate also support this suspicion. In this patient, the clinical pattern is most consistent with that of Wegener's granulomatosis (see Table 6-6).

2. The presence of WBC casts suggests interstitial nephritis as a possible etiology. Acute pyelonephritis or acute allergic interstitial nephritis resulting from the use of one of the multiple antibiotics are other possible diagnoses. The absence of rash and eosinophilia tend to exclude the latter. Pyelonephritis can be excluded by urine and blood cultures. The presence of RBC casts suggests GN of the nephritic or rapidly progressive variety. Nevertheless, the multisystem nature of this woman's disease as well as the evidence of interstitial nephritis would make one consider vasculitis more likely.

This case demonstrates the overlap in clinical features typical of renal vascular diseases. Because the patient has definite evidence of both interstitial and glomerular disease, renal vasculitis is a primary concern.

3. Although the renal biopsy is rarely diagnostic when performed in patients with vasculitis, it does provide useful information. This patient's renal biopsy showed marked interstitial inflammation with acute inflammatory cells including lymphocytes, plasmacytes, and polymorphonuclear cells. Eosinophils were not prominent. The interstitial inflammation had a granulomatous appearance in some areas, although no obvious granulomata were seen. The glomeruli were hypercellular with segmental necrosis. No deposits were seen on electron microscopy, and immunofluorescence studies showed nonspecific staining for fibrin. The walls of the arteries and arterioles were distorted by fragmentation of the elastic lamellas, and fibrin deposition was suggested.

These biopsy findings are typical, although not diagnostic, of Wegener's granulomatosis. Similar findings may be seen with polyarteritis nodosa or, indeed, with RPGN without systemic disease. Recently, the question has been raised whether or not these forms of idiopathic RPGN are, in fact, a "limited" variety of Wegener's granulomatosis. Determination of the recently described antineutrophilcyloplasmic antibody (ANCA) may distinguish these from idiopathic RPGN.

4. Corticosteroids and cyclophosphamide are indicated for patients with Wegener's granulomatosis, polyarteritis nodosa, and ANCA-positive RPGN without immune deposits.

References

Balow JE. Renal vasculitis. Kidney Int 1985; 27:954–964.

Case records of the Massachusetts General Hospital. (Case 11-1982): Chronic urticaria, proteinuria, and cryglobulinemia. N Engl J Med 1982; 306:657–668.

Falk RJ, Jennette JC. Anti-neutrophilic cytoplasma autoantibodies with specificity for myeloperoxidase in patients with systemic vasculitis and idiopathic necrotizing and cresentic glomerulonephritis. N Engl J Med 1988; 318:1651–1657.

Fauci AS, Haynes BF, Katz P. The spectrum of vasculitis: clinical, pathologic, immunologic, and therapeutic considerations. Ann Int Med 1978; 89:660–676.

Fauci AS, Haynes BS, Katz P, Wolff SM. Wegener's granulomatosis: prospective clinical and therapeutic experience with 85 patients for 21 years. Ann Int Med 1983; 98:76–85.

Jacobson HR. Ischemic renal disease: an overlooked clinical entity? Kidney Int 1988; 34:729–743.

Kasiske B. Relationship between vascular disease and age-associated changes in the human kidney. Kidney Int 1987; 31:1153–1159.

Lessman RK, Johnson SK, Coburn JW, Kaufman J. Renal artery embolism: clinical features and long-term follow-up of 17 cases. Ann Int Med 1978; 89:477–482.

Llach F, Papper S, Massry SG. The clinical spectrum of renal vein thrombosis: acute and chronic. Am J Med 1980; 69:819–827.

McGowan JA, Greenberg A. Cholesterol atheroembolic renal disease. Am J Nephrol 1986; 6:135–139.

Novick AL, Pohl MA, Schreiber M, et al. Revascularization for preservation of renal function in patients with atherosclerotic renovascular disease. J Urol 1983; 129:907–912.

7 Clinical Disorders of Sodium Balance: Derangements of the Extracellular Volume

- Case Presentations

- Control of Sodium Balance

- Disorders of Body Sodium (ECV) Depletion

- Diagnostic and Therapeutic Approach to Patients with Body Sodium Depletion

- Disorders of Body Sodium Excess (Edematous Disorders)

- Treatment of the Edematous Patient

- Diagnostic Approach to Patients with Edema

- Case Discussions

Case 7-1

A 44-year-old man presented with a 4- to 5-day history of fever, myalgia, nausea, vomiting, and diarrhea.

Physical examination showed him to be alert and oriented. His weight was 70 kg, his pulse rate was 108 beats per minute, and his blood pressure was 134/80 and 106/60 with the patient in the supine and sitting positions, respectively. No neck veins were detected despite his supine position. There was no edema.

Laboratory evaluation revealed sodium of 138 mEq/L, potassium of 3.4 mEq/L, chloride of 94 mEq/L, and bicarbonate of 30 mEq/L. The BUN was 30 mg/dl, and creatinine was 1.2 mg/dl.

Questions

1. What would you expect the urinary sodium concentration to be?
2. What fluid replacement should he receive?
3. How much fluid should he receive?

Case 7-2

A 74-year-old man with Milroy's disease (congenital lymphedema) presented to the emergency room after an episode of postural syncope. He had recently lost 8 to 10 lb—a weight loss that was attributed to nausea and anorexia.

Physical examination showed him to be mildly lethargic, well-oriented, and without focal neurologic deficit. He had dry mucous membranes, no rales but marked firm, nonpitting peripheral edema. His blood pressure was 164/82 and 108/70 in the sitting and standing positions, respectively. Pulse rose from 88 to 104 beats per minute on standing.

Laboratory work showed that the serum sodium was 130 mEq/L, potassium was 2.4 mEq/L, chloride was 94 mEq/L and bicarbonate was 30 mEq/L. His BUN was 28 mg/dl, and his creatinine was 1.3 mg/dl.

Questions

1. Is his total body sodium high or low?
2. What medication do you suspect he was taking?
3. What do you believe his urinary sodium concentration was initially and 12 hours later?
4. What would be the appropriate therapy for this patient?

Case 7-3

A 64-year-old man was hospitalized with shortness of breath and progressive edema. Past history was positive for long-standing hypertension and a previous myocardial infarction. He was taking no medicines at the time of admission.

Physical examination showed jugular venous distention (10 cm H_2O), bilateral pulmonary rales, 2+ pitting peripheral edema, and an S_3 gallop. Blood pressure was 122/76.

Laboratory evaluations showed the following: serum sodium was 134 mEq/L, potassium was 4 mEq/L, chloride was 98 mEq/L, and bicarbonate was 24 mEq/L. Urinalysis showed specific gravity of 1.026, and trace protein. Urine sodium was 10 mEq/L, BUN was 18 mg/dl, and creatinine was 0.8 mg/dl.

Questions

1. What is the cause of his edema?
2. What is the appropriate therapy?

Case 7-4

A 58-year-old woman was readmitted to the hospital for chest pain and shortness of breath. One month earlier, she underwent coronary artery bypass grafting for angina. Her postoperative course was complicated by heart failure. She was discharged 1 week before readmission, and was taking furosemide (80 mg twice per day), digoxin, nitrates, and hydralazine at that time.

Physical findings were 1+ edema, bilateral rales, and jugular venous distention. Her blood pressure was 118/70.

She was treated with bedrest, salt restriction, and oxygen, and her dose of furosemide was increased to 120 mg twice per day. On Day 3, she began receiving captopril, as well. Results of the laboratory tests for Days 1 through 8 are shown in the following table.

	Day 1	Day 3	Day 5	Day 8
Weight	56.0 kg	54.0 kg	55.0 kg	55.0 kg
Na	125.0 mEq/L	124.0 mEq/L	126.0 mEq/L	125.0 mEq/L
K	4.0 mEq/L	3.8 mEq/L	4.2 mEq/L	5.4 mEq/L
Cl	85.0 mEq/L	85.0 mEq/L	84.0 mEq/L	83.0 mEq/L
HCO_3	27.0 mEq/L	28.0 mEq/L	24.0 mEq/L	20.0 mEq/L
BUN	42.0 mg/dl	54.0 mg/dl	62.0 mg/dl	94.0 mg/dl
Creatinine	1.5 mg/dl	1.8 mg/dl	2.2 mg/dl	5.0 mg/dl

Questions

1. What is the cause of the azotemia on Day 1 and the worsening of azotemia on Days 3 and 5?
2. What treatment should be administered on Day 5?
3. How could one have avoided this situation?

Case 7-5

A 57-year-old man was admitted to the hospital for dyspnea, vomiting, weakness, and a progressive increase in edema and abdominal girth. He denied having had previous heart problems, hypertension, proteinuria, liver disease, or a history of alcohol abuse.

On examination, his blood pressure was 98/62, and his sclerae were icteric. He had marked jugular venous distention, ascites, and peripheral and sacral edema. Spider angiomata were evident on the chest wall. Liver span was 10 cm. Stool was hemocult positive, and serial sevens were done poorly. Urinalysis demonstrated a trace protein with an SG of 1.024. The laboratory values are shown in the following table.

Na	128.0 mEq/L
K	3.4 mEq/L
Cl	98.0 mEq/L
HCO$_3$	24.0 mEq/L
Bilirubin	4.3 mg/dl
Albumin	28.0 mg/dl
BUN	7.0 mg/dl
Creatinine	0.8 mg/dl
Urinary Na	6 mEq/L

Questions

1. What is the cause of the edema?
2. What IV fluids should be initiated?
3. What is the appropriate treatment?

Changes in the extracellular fluid volume parallel changes in total body sodium. Therefore, excesses or deficiencies in total body sodium are reflected clinically by findings of ECV overload or deficit. A derangement in ECV is best detected by the physical examination, with the clinician searching for the presence or absence of rales, edema, jugular venous distention, third heart sound (S_3) gallop, dry mucous membranes, and orthostatic hypotension. Total body sodium has no direct relationship to the serum sodium concentration ([Na]). *The serum [Na] is therefore useless when defining abnormalities of total body sodium (ECV).*

Derangements in sodium balance can result from changes in salt intake, gastrointestinal losses, and most importantly, changes in the renal handling of sodium. Before discussing the clinical disorders of salt balance, however, we will examine the factors controlling the renal regulation of sodium.

Control of Sodium Balance

The kidneys control sodium balance by adjusting renal excretion to sodium intake. Figure 7-1 depicts the sodium balance of an individual who abruptly increases dietary sodium intake by 150 mEq daily. Over the next few days, the patient will have positive sodium balance, gaining approximately 1 kg of body weight. However, sodium excretion will gradually increase over this same period until it equals dietary intake (150 mEq/day) and the patient achieves a new steady state where output equals intake and body weight is stable. If dietary intake decreases abruptly, a period of negative sodium balance and weight loss occurs until renal conservation of sodium cuts urinary losses so that they are again equal to the dietary intake of sodium. Several factors are recognized as critical to this renal regulation of sodium balance (Table 7-1).

Glomerular filtration rate was the first factor recognized as contributing to renal sodium balance. An increase in GFR increases the filtered load of sodium and tends to augment excretion, whereas decrements in GFR decrease sodium excretion. However, sodium excretion is the sum of the sodium filtered minus the sodium reabsorbed by the tubules. Because of the factors controlling reabsorption of filtered sodium, one rarely sees a clinical derangement of sodium balance caused solely by changes in GFR. One exception, of

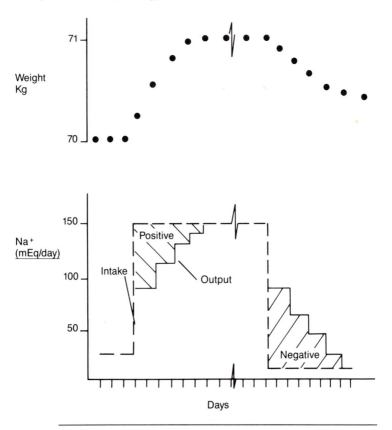

Figure 7-1: Normal sodium balance. Changes in dietary sodium are reflected by changes in urinary sodium and body weight.

course, is severe renal failure, where the GFR and thus the filtered sodium load approaches zero. On the other hand, changes in GFR (and in particular, the individual factors controlling GFR) significantly influence sodium reabsorption in the proximal tubule and thus contribute to the pathophysiology of most sodium-retaining states.

Four factors determine the GFR:

1. Renal blood flow (RBF).
2. The hydrostatic pressure gradient across the glomerular capillary (GC) (abbreviated here H_{GC}).
3. The oncotic (π) pressure gradient across the GC π_{GC}).
4. The permeability (K_f) of the glomerular capillary wall.

Of these four factors, alterations in RBF and H_{GC} commonly contribute to deranged sodium balance by affecting both filtered load and tubular absorption.

The mineralocorticoid *aldosterone* was the second major factor shown to significantly influence sodium balance. Aldosterone stimulates renal tubular reabsorption of sodium in exchange for potassium or hydrogen. Aldosterone (or its synthetic counterpart deoxycorticosterone acetate [DOCA]) thus promotes renal sodium (volume) retention and weight-gain (positive sodium balance). The sodium retention is finite, however. Within a few days, sodium excretion returns to normal, once again equalling intake. The patient is in a new state of sodium balance with a steady body weight (albeit approximately 1 kg greater than the original weight). This ability to overcome the effects of the mineralocorticoid by increasing sodium excretion is termed the "mineralocorticoid escape." The effects of exogenously administered mineralocorticoid and this "escape" phenomenon are depicted in Figure 7-2.

In 1961, deWardener and colleagues demonstrated that an ani-

Table 7-1 Factors Controlling Renal Sodium Excretion

Glomerular filtration rate

Aldosterone

"Third factors"
    Renin angiotensin system
    Peritubular Starling forces
    Atrial natriuretic factor
    Norepinephrine
    Prostaglandins (PGE_2)
    Kallikreinin-kinins
    Antidiuretic hormone
    Intrarenal redistribution of blood flow

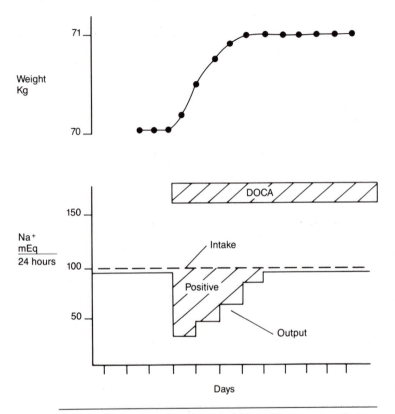

Figure 7-2: Excess mineralocorticoid (DOCA) causes transient sodium retention and persistent weight gain in normal individuals. Within days, however, sodium excretion and sodium balance return to normal, a phenomenon known as mineralocorticoid "escape."

mal with decreased GFR (caused by aortic obstruction) and excess mineralocorticoid exogenously administered was still able to excrete a sodium load. This classic experiment suggested a "*third factor*" controlling renal sodium excretion (Fig. 7-3). In fact, there are several other "third" factors known to influence renal sodium

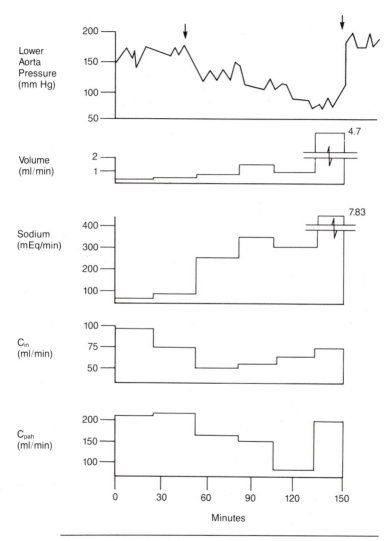

Lower Aorta Pressure (mm Hg)

Volume (ml/min)

Sodium (mEq/min)

C_{in} (ml/min)

C_{pah} (ml/min)

Minutes

Figure 7-3: The deWardener experiment demonstrating a natriuresis occurring in saline-loaded dogs despite low GFR and excess mineralocorticoid indicating that a "third" factor (or factors) contributes to the control of sodium excretion.

handling (see Table 7-1). Understanding the influence of these factors is perhaps best accomplished by examining segmental renal tubular sodium reabsorption (Fig. 7-4).

Of the approximate 150 L of filtered saline daily (110 ml/minute × 1,440 minutes/day), 60 to 75% is reabsorbed both actively and passively by proximal tubular segments. Norepinephrine released from renal nerve-endings appears to stimulate proximal sodium absorption directly. The passive sodium reabsorption in this segment is largely dependent on peritubular Starling forces—that is, the net differences in hydrostatic and oncotic (π) pressure between the peritubular capillary (PTC) and proximal tubular lumen (H_{PTC} and π_{PTC}, respectively). When the H_{PTC} is low and/or the π_{PTC} is high, proximal reabsorption of filtered sodium is increased.

One of the major determinants of both H_{PTC} and π_{PTC} is the tone of the glomerular efferent arteriolar sphincter (ES). Constriction of the ES lowers H_{PTC}. It also raises π_{PTC} by increasing the glomerular hydrostatic pressure (H_{GC}) and filtration of protein-free fluid. Plasma proteins are thus concentrated along the course of the glomerular capillary, which directly increases the π_{PTC}. This effect of ES constriction influencing glomerular and peritubular Starling forces is demonstrated in Figure 7-5.

ES constriction is largely mediated by angiotensin II (AII). Thus conditions associated with excess AII, such as a decreased ECV (e.g., severe vomiting or diarrhea) or decreased "effective" ECV (e.g., congestive heart failure), are characterized by enhanced proximal tubular reabsorption of filtered sodium due in part to the effect of ES constriction on peritubular Starling forces. Other factors contributing to the avid sodium retention of these patients include increased aldosterone, norepinephrine (both circulating

---

Figure 7-4: *A*, Elements of renal sodium excretion according to ➤ filtration and active ($\rightarrow$), passive ($\dashrightarrow$), and coupled (0) sodium reabsorption. *B*, The table below identifies the factors (and their modifiers) known to control sodium handling in each segment.

AS = afferent arteriolar sphincter; ES = efferent arteriolar sphincter; K_f = glomerular capillary permeability; H = hydrostatic pressure; π = oncotic pressure; ANP = atrial natriuretic peptide; ADH = antidiuretic hormone.

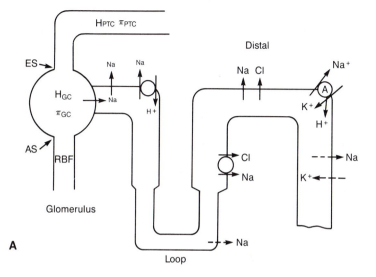

A

B

	Filtration (GFR)	Reabsorption				Excretion
		Proxmial Tubule	Loop	Distal Tubule	Collecting Tubule	
mEq/day	21,000	15,500	2,100	2,100	1,050.0	210.0
Vol(L/day)	150	111	15	15	7.5	1.5
% Filtrate	100	74	10	10	5.0	1.0
Controlling Factors	RBF H_{GC} π_{GC} K_f	Norepi H_{PTC} π_{PTC}	Cl absorption PGE_2 ADH	Unknown	Aldo (A) ANP PGE_2 ADH	
Increased by	Low ECV ANP Dopamine High cardiac output	Low ECV A_{II}	Low ECV NSAID	Low ECV	Low ECV NSAID Aldosterone	
Decreased by	Low ECV NSAID Low cardiac output	Acetazola-mide Mannitol ACE inhibitors	Furosemide Bumetamide Ethacrynic acid	Thiazides Chlorhali-done Metalozone	Spironolac-tone Triamterene Amiloride	

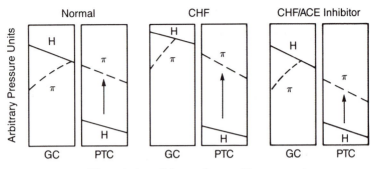

Figure 7-5: Approximate glomerular and peritubular capillary hydrostatic (H) and oncotic (π) pressure profiles in normals, patients with CHF, and patients with CHF treated with ACE inhibitors. The solid arrows ($\rightarrow$) indicate the net driving force for proximal tubular sodium reabsorption. Constriction of the efferent arteriolar sphincter by AII raises the H_{GC}, thus increasing proximal tubular sodium reabsorption. These pressures (and therefore sodium reabsorption) return towards normal when AII inhibition causes ES relaxation.

and released from renal nerves), and antidiuretic hormone which appears to have a small influence on sodium reabsorption. These latter factors appear to stimulate sodium reabsorption in more distal nephron segments.

Approximately 10% of filtered sodium is reabsorbed in the ascending loop of Henle, largely driven by active chloride reabsorption. Prostaglandins (particularly PGE_2) appear to effect a natriuresis in the loop (as well as in the collecting tubule), partially explaining the sodium retention so commonly noted with nonsteroidal anti-inflammatory drugs. Approximately 10% of glomerular filtrate is reabsorbed by the early distal convoluted tubule. An additional 6 to 8% is absorbed by the cortical collecting tubule (late distal tubule). Here, sodium reabsorption (in exchange for potassium and hydrogen) is largely driven by aldosterone.

The net result of the reabsoption in the tubular segments is a 99% fractional reabsorption of filtered sodium (1% fractional excretion of sodium [$FE_{NA} = 1\%$]) in normal individuals. With a decrease in actual or effective ECV, however, the FE_{NA} can decrease to far less than 1%.

Disorders of Body Sodium (ECV) Depletion

Sodium-depleted states are detected clinically by a decrease in the ECV. The typical signs, symptoms, and laboratory values of ECV depletion are shown in Table 7-2. Of these, tachycardia, postural hypotension, and the urine chemistries are the most reliable. Although Table 7-2 reflects an attempt to categorize the findings according to mild, moderate, or severe deficiencies in the ECV, the astute clinician will remember that significant overlap occurs. In particular, the rapidity with which the derangement occurs can affect the symptoms and physical findings—amplifying them if the derangement develops rapidly, and dampening them if its development is slow.

Table 7-2 Signs and Symptoms of Total Body Sodium (ECV) Depletion Expressed as the Percentage of Total Body Water Lost

Loss	Symptoms	Signs	Laboratory Findings
Mild (5% TBW)	Thirst Weakness Fatigue	Dry mucous membranes Dark urine	↑ Urine SG ↑ Urine OSM ↑ Hematocrit ↓ Urine Na
Moderate (10% TBW)	Headache Anorexia Nausea Cramping Postural dizziness	Resting tachycardia Flat neck veins Oliguria Orthostatic hypotension	↑ BUN ↑ BUN: Creatinine ↑ Phosphorus ↑ Uric acid
Severe (15% TBW)	Apathy Lethargy Confusion	Hypotension Hypothermia	↑ Creatinine Leukocytosis

SG = specific gravity; OSM = osmolarity.

Mild, moderate, and severe depletion of total body sodium are here defined as percentages of the total body water (TBW) (approximately 60% of total body weight). These percentages can also be used to calculate the volume of replacement fluid. Thus, a 70-kg patient with symptoms and signs of moderate ECV depletion should receive approximately 4,200 ml of isotonic saline as replacement (70 kg × 60% = 42L of TBW × 10% = 4.2 L).

ECV depletion results from *sodium loss,* usually via the gastrointestinal tract or kidneys (Table 7-3). Gastrointestinal losses are the most common. Skin losses alone rarely account for significant ECV depletion, with the exception of severe burns and extensive dermatologic disease. Sequestration of volume into a "third space" may compromise the intravascular volume, even though actual total ECV is unchanged.

Renal sodium losses result from a failure of the renal tubules to appropriately reabsorb filtered sodium. Diuretics are the most common cause of renal salt-wasting, but occasionally renal parenchymal

Table 7-3 Causes of Total Body Sodium (ECV) Depletion

Extrarenal Sodium Loss
  Gastrointestinal
    Vomiting/gastric suction
    Small bowel fistula
    Diarrhea
  Skin
    Heat
    Burns
    Severe dermatitis
  Third space
    Crush injuries
    Small bowel obstruction
    Peritonitis
    Pancreatitis

Renal Sodium Loss
  Diuretics
  "Salt-losing" nephropathies
  Hypoaldosteronism
  Bartter's syndrome
  Renal tubular acidosis

disease (particularly interstitial nephritis) can also cause salt loss. Distal tubular salt loss accompanies hypoaldosteronism regardless of its etiology (see Chapter 9). Renal tubular acidosis (RTA) causes sodium bicarbonaturia (see Chapter 10).

Diagnostic and Therapeutic Approach to Patients with Body Sodium Depletion

A diagnostic approach to patients with total body sodium depletion is outlined in Figure 7-6. First, hemorrhage should be excluded by history, physical examination, and documentation of a hematocrit of less than 40%. One should remember that in a volume-contracted patient (one with low ECV), blood loss can be masked by hemoconcentration.

After hemorrhage has been excluded, the urinary sodium should distinguish the renal sodium waster from a patient with extrarenal sodium loss. If the kidney is the source of sodium loss, the urinary sodium will be greater than 20 mEq/L in a volume-contracted patient. If, on the other hand, salt loss has occurred via the intestinal tract, the urinary sodium will be less than 10 mEq/L. If the patient has chronic azotemia, the urinary sodium may not fall to this level.

The most common causes of gastrointestinal and renal salt loss are associated with either acidosis or alkalosis, further aiding the differential diagnosis. Thus, metabolic acidosis (serum HCO_3 <24 mEq/L) in a renal sodium waster suggests RTA, hypoaldosteronism, or some underlying renal disease, usually interstitial nephritis ("salt-losing nephropathy"). Metabolic alkalosis (serum HCO_3 >27 mEq/L), on the other hand, accompanies Bartter's syndrome or diuretics. Similarly, when extrarenal sodium loss is documented (urinary sodium <20 mEq/L), metabolic acidosis suggests loss of lower gastrointestinal fluid rich in bicarbonate, whereas metabolic alkalosis suggests loss of the acidic gastric contents.

Therapeutically, patients with sodium depletion need sodium repletion, usually via isotonic salt solutions. Table 7-4 shows the typical daily volume and electrolyte composition of body fluids likely to account for sodium depletion. These values serve as a guide to replacement fluid management. The patient with sodium deple-

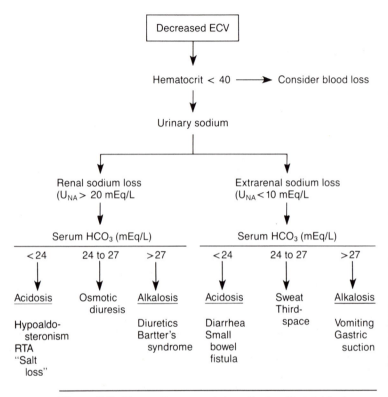

Figure 7-6: Diagnostic approach to patients with total body sodium (ECV) depletion.

tion (ECV contraction) from vomiting needs replacement with normal saline intravenously. (Concomitant renal loss of potassium resulting from secondary hyperaldosteronism usually necessitates the addition of potassium, as well). In the patient with severe diarrhea, where colonic fluid is relatively rich in potassium and bicarbonate, these electrolytes are added to the replacement fluids. Sweat is essentially devoid of electrolytes and requires replacement of water only. Replacement of urinary losses is highly variable,

Table 7-4 Composition of Lost Fluids Typically Responsible for Total Body Sodium (ECV) Depletion*

Fluid Lost	Volume (L/day)†	Composition (mEq/L)				Replacement Fluid
		Na	K	Cl	HCO₃	
Gastric	0–2	60–110‡	10	120	0	NS
Small bowel	0–3	140	10	120	30	NS
Colon	0.5–4.0	120	30	90	60	0.45% NS, KCl, NaHCO₃
Skin	0.1–0.8	40	0	0	0	D₅W
Urine§	0–5 +	50	40	90	0	0.45% NS, KCl

*Recommended replacement fluid and electrolytes should approximate that of fluid lost.
†Range from physiologic to pathologic.
‡At gastric pH < 4, Na = 60; at gastric pH > 4, Na = 110.
§Numbers approximate physiologic conditions. Urine composition can vary considerably depending on drugs and/or disease.
NaHCO₃ = sodium bicarbonate; NS = normal saline; D₅W = 5% dextrose in water.

depending on the use of diuretics or type and extent of renal disease. When sodium loss occurs through the urine, direct measurement of the patient's urinary electrolytes is the best guide to therapy.

The composition of the common IV replacement solution is shown in Table 7-5. Therapeutic replacement therefore becomes a

Table 7-5 Composition of Typical Crystalloid Replacement Solution

Solution	mOsm/L	Composition (mEq/L)			
		Na	K	Cl	HCO₃*
D₅W	0	0	0	0	0
0.45% NS	155	77	0	77	0
0.9% NS	310	154	0	154	0
Ringer's lactate	275	130	4	109	28*
Hypertonic saline (3%)	1,025	513	0	513	0

*Lactate converted to HCO₃ in liver.
NS = normal saline; D₅W = 5% dextrose in water.

matter of simple arithmetic as one estimates the volume and electrolyte composition of the fluid lost and adds to it the expected maintenance fluid and electrolytes for the next 24 hours. This can then be administered to the patient at an appropriate rate according to his or her clinical status.

Disorders of Body Sodium Excess (Edematous Disorders)

The major edematous disorders (disorders of excess total body sodium) are listed in Table 7-6 with the mechanism(s) primarily responsible for the sodium excess in each case. Because of the kidney's enormous capacity to excrete excess salt, excessive oral intake alone rarely accounts for edema. However, rapid saline and/or sodium bicarbonate administration during resuscitation of the critically ill can occasionally produce this syndrome.

Acute or chronic renal failure from any cause is often associated with edema as sodium intake exceeds its glomerular filtration. At a GFR of 5 ml/min (7.2 L/day), the filtered load of sodium is 1,008 mEq (7.2 L × 140 mEq/L). Even if the fractional excretion of sodium is 10% (exceedingly high) only 100 mEq of sodium would be excreted daily. Dietary intake exceeding 100 mEq of sodium (2,300

Table 7-6 Causes of Excess Total Body Sodium and the Pathophysiologic Mechanisms Responsible for Sodium Retention in each Case

Cause	Intake of Na	↓ GFR	↑ Aldosteronism	"Third factors"
Excess intake	X			
Renal failure		X		
Hyperaldosteronism			X	
Heart failure		X	X	X
Cirrhosis		X	X	X
Nephrotic syndrome		X	X	X

mg) daily would thus result in excess total body sodium and eventually edema formation.

Primary hyperaldosteronism is recognized clinically by hypertension and occasionally by edema. The edema is rarely severe because of the "mineralocorticoid escape" phenomenon described earlier. Other sequelae of excess aldosterone are hypokalemia and metabolic alkalosis, which result from renal tubular loss of potassium and hydrogen, respectively. Whereas primary hyperaldosteronism is exceedingly rare, secondary hyperaldosteronism caused by low effective ECV often contributes to the renal sodium retention of *heart failure, cirrhosis,* and *nephrotic syndrome.*

Figures 7-7 through 7-9 outline the pathogenetic mechanisms responsible for the renal sodium retention and edema formation that occur with *heart failure, cirrhosis, and nephrosis,* respectively. Despite their differences, the primary disorder causing each of these syndromes appears to be a low effective circulating volume. This decreased "effective volume" stimulates various mechanisms such as the sympathetic nervous system and renin-angiotensin-aldosterone system, resulting in renal sodium retention.

Treatment of the Edematous Patient

Based on this pathophysiology, one can devise a rational approach to treatment. First, because edematous patients are by definition overloaded with total body sodium, all should be placed on sodium restriction. In this setting, the importance of sodium restriction (with the patient receiving no more than 500 to 1,500 mg of sodium per day) cannot be overemphasized.

Increasing the effective blood volume is next in importance. For the patient with heart failure, this requires that cardiac output be improved by correcting known mechanical factors, controlling afterload (vasodilators), optimizing left ventricular end-diastolic volume (nitrates, diuretics), and maximizing myocardial function (inotropes). In this regard, ACE inhibitors appear to have special value. These agents not only serve as vasodilators but also alter intrarenal hemodynamics. By decreasing efferent arteriolar sphincter pressure, ACE inhibitors lower the glomerular capillary hy-

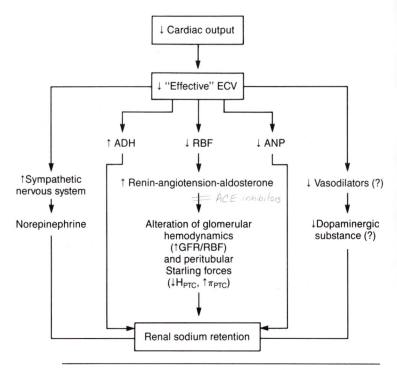

Figure 7-7: Pathophysiologic schema indicating some of the factors involved in the renal sodium retention that occurs with CHF.

drostatic pressure (H_{GC}) and the fraction of RBF that is filtered (filtration fraction), resulting in higher H_{PTC} and lower π_{PTC} (see Fig. 7-5). The net result is a decrease in proximal tubular sodium reabsorption and an improved natriuresis and water diuresis (see Chapter 8).

In patients with cirrhosis, intrahepatic factors may lead to activation of sympathetic or renin angiotensin systems. Effective circulating volume is also compromised in these patients, leading to renal sodium retention, as in the case of patients with heart failure.

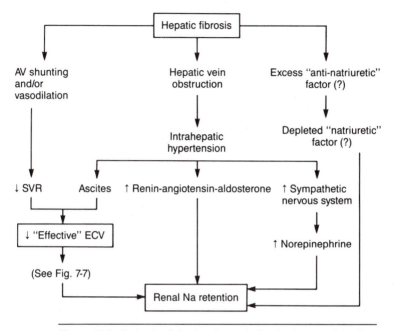

Figure 7-8: Pathophysiologic schema indicating some of the factors involved in the renal sodium retention that occurs with cirrhosis.

SVR = systemic vascular resistance; AV = arteriovenous.

Without first improving liver function, correction of this compromised effective volume is very difficult. Slow, continuous shunting of peritoneal fluid to the venous circulation (LeVeen's shunt, Denver shunt) holds promise for some patients with refractory ascites and renal dysfunction.

In nephrotic and some malnourished patients, hypoalbuminemia is the major factor contributing to a low effective circulating volume. The mechanisms promoting renal sodium retention are similar to those in heart failure and cirrhosis. Primary therapy to increase effective volume in nephrotics must therefore be directed at diminishing urinary protein loss. Specific therapy based on renal histology

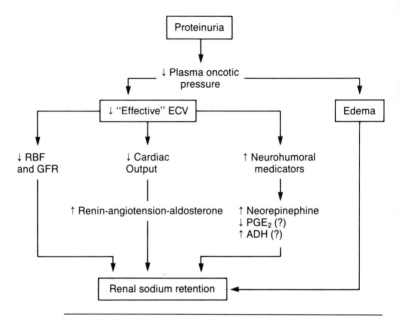

Figure 7-9: Pathophysiologic schema indicating some of the factors involved in the renal sodium retention that occurs with nephrotic syndrome.

is sometimes helpful (see Chapter 4). Nonspecific therapy includes ACE inhibitors, low-protein diets, and nonsteroidal anti-inflammatory drugs, all of which appear to diminish urinary protein loss quantitatively. Close monitoring of serum creatinine is always necessary when administering these drugs to edematous patients.

Diuretics are an important adjunct to therapy for edematous patients. However, when treating disorders of decreased effective volume, one must be mindful of the diuretics' potential for toxicity. For example, in patients with congestive heart failure whose renal function deteriorates while they are undergoing ACE inhibitor therapy, overdiuresis often appears to be responsible. As in the case of the hypothetical patients of Table 7-7, diuretics may "fix" renal blood flow at a critically low level, mandating a decrement in GFR

Table 7-7 Possible Mechanism to Explain the Deterioration in GFR Often Noted in Severe Heart Failure Patients When Given an ACE Inhibitor

	Pre-ACE Inhibitor			Post-ACE Inhibitor	
	Normal Individual	Patient A	Patient B	Patient A	Patient B
Cardiac Index (CI) (L/min/m^2)	3	1.8	1.8	2.2	1.8
RBF (ml/min)	600	100	75	180	75
H_{GC} (mm Hg)	20	24	24	16	16
GFR (ml/min)	120	25	25	30	12
GFR:RBF (filtration fraction)	0.20	0.25	0.33	0.16	0.16

Hypothetical Patient A (no longer receiving diuretics) and Patient B (receiving diuretics) have identical CI and baseline GFR. Patient A responds to ACE inhibition by increasing RBF, thus offsetting the fall in H_{GC}. GFR improves because of improved RBF. In Patient B, however, the RBF is relatively "fixed" because of diuretics, such that GFR is more dependent on H_{GC}. A decrease in H_{GC} after ACE inhibition thus results in a marked fall in GFR.

when H_{GC} is decreased by efferent arteriolar sphincter relaxation (because of ACE inhibition). In this regard, some patients with heart failure (those with highly compromised and static RBF while receiving diuretics) are similar to patients with bilateral renal artery stenosis whose renal function often deteriorates with ACE inhibitor therapy (and usually with diuretic therapy). Therefore, before initiating ACE inhibitor therapy in azotemic or hyponatremic patients with heart failure, one should consider discontinuing or decreasing diuretics.

Figure 7-4 outlines the common diuretics according to their primary site of action. There is very little therapeutic difference between drugs with the same site of action. When multiple diuretics are necessary to effect a diuresis, drugs with different sites of action are best combined. Acetazolamide is particularly useful with a loop diuretic in patients with heart failure when fractional proximal reabsorption is increased. In patients with cirrhosis, loop diuretics are often too potent and may precipitate a marked decline in renal function. Generally, renal function will remain stable in cirrhotic patients if the net fluid loss is less than 750 ml/day (the approximate capacity to mobilize ascitic fluid). For these patients, a combination of agents with more distal sites of action, such as a thiazide and spironolactone combination, is more appropriate—although it should be remembered that ascites per se is not an indication to initiate diuretic therapy. Avoidance of vigorous diuresis (>1 to 2 kg/day) or paracentesis (>1 L/day) and very judicious use of NSAIDs are mandatory when one is treating patients with cirrhosis. One must also remember that the collecting tubule diuretics can be potassium-sparing only if urine flow is suppressed by low sodium intake. Again, salt restriction is the primary therapy for the edematous disorders.

Diagnostic Approach to Patients with Edema

The characteristic laboratory and physical findings of the edematous disorders are outlined in Table 7-8. Usually, distinctive laboratory and physical abnormalities easily differentiate these patients. For example, a markedly elevated BUN and creatinine level is seen with renal failure, marked proteinuria (greater than 3.5 g/day) with nephrotic syndrome, and hyperbilirubinemia and abnormal liver function tests are seen with cirrhosis. Hypertension is the hallmark of primary hyperaldosteronism, with hypokalemia and metabolic alkalosis the typical laboratory features (when the patient is no longer receiving diuretics). Although numerous biochemical derangements are common with CHF, the physical examination remains the best test for distinguishing patients with CHF from those with other edematous disorders (i.e., other causes of ECV overload and edema).

These physical and laboratory findings support a diagnostic algorithm (Fig. 7-10) for approaching the patient with total body sodium excess. First, renal failure is identified by severe azotemia. The absence of hypertension, hypokalemic alkalosis, and sometimes hypernatremia virtually exclude the diagnosis of hyperaldosteronism. Nephrotic-range proteinuria and hypoalbuminemia distinguish

Table 7-8. Laboratory and Physical Findings Helpful in the Differential Diagnosis of the Edematous Disorders

Laboratory Findings	Renal Failure	Hyper-aldosteronism	CHF	Cirrhosis	Nephrotic Syndrome
Hematocrit	↓	N	N	↓	N
BUN	↑*	N	↑	N–↓	N
Creatinine	↑*	N	N	N	N
BUN:Creatinine	10	10	15	5	5
Serum Na	N–↓	N–↑	N–↓	N–↓	N–↓
Serum K	N–↑	↓	N	N–↓	N
Albumin	N–↓	N	N	↓*	↓
Bilirubin	N	N	N–↑	↑	N
Cholesterol	N	N	N	N	↑
Urine Na (mEq/L)	> 30	> 50	< 20	< 20	< 20
Urine osmolarity (mOsm/L)	300	300	> 450	> 450	> 450
Urine protein (g/day)	< 3	N	N	N	> 3*
Blood pressure	N–↑	↑↑*	N	N	N
Physical examination	Asterixis Pericardial rub Edema	Edema (±)	S₃* JVD Rales ↓ Carotid pulse N–↑ Liver Edema	Jaundice Prominent ascites Spider angiomata Fetor N–↓ Liver Marked asterixis	Edema

*The most reliable test for the disorder. N = normal; ↑ = increased; ↓ = decreased; N–↑ = normal to increased; S₃ = third heart sound; JVD = jugular venous distention.

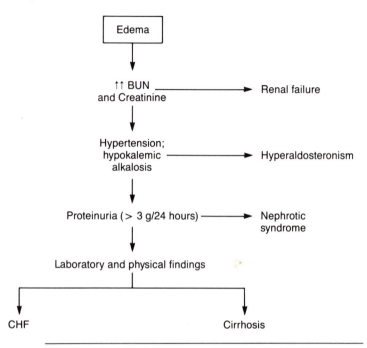

Figure 7-10: Diagnostic approach to patients with edema (total body sodium excess).

the nephrotic syndrome. Finally, the physical examination and history will differentiate cirrhosis from CHF (see Table 7-8).

Case 7-1: *Discussion*

1. This patient presents with obvious ECV depletion as determined by the physical examination. The resting tachycardia and orthostatic hypotension are suggestive of at least a 10% loss of total body volume.

The urine sodium is usually less than 10 mEq/L in patients with ECV depletion caused by extrarenal causes. FE_{NA} should be less than 1%. The BUN:creatinine ratio is approximately 20:1. These values are all expected findings in this patient.

2. Isotonic fluid administration is indicated in this patient. Normal saline with potassium chloride would be the appropriate IV fluid.

3. To replace a 10% ECV loss in a 70-kg man, approximately 4,200 ml is required (60% of 70 kg = 42 L TBW × 10% = 4.2 L).

Case 7-2: *Discussion*

1. The results of this patient's physical examination are somewhat confusing. Despite signs of ECV depletion (the orthostatic tachycardia, hypotension, and dry mucous membranes) he had edema. The edema was nonpitting, however, and likely caused by the Milroy's disease. His total body sodium (volume) is likely increased (i.e., high) but his intravascular volume is decreased.

2. His doctor had made the mistake of treating his inaccessible lymphedema with furosemide. Depletion of the ECV then occurred, accounting for his orthostatic syncope. His hypokalemia and metabolic alkalosis are other clues that he was taking diuretics.

3. If the patient had recently taken furosemide, his urinary sodium might be high (>20 mEq/L). As the drug effect wears off, however, urine sodium should decrease to less than 10 mEq/L; FE_{NA} should be less than 1%.

4. The furosemide should be discontinued, and cautious replacement of isotonic saline and potassium chloride should be initiated. Over the long-term, his edema should be treated with measured compression stockings and dietary sodium restriction.

Case 7-3: *Discussion*

1. The cause of this man's edema is probably heart failure. Primary hyperaldosteronism is unlikely without hypertension or hypokalemic alkalosis. The normal BUN and creatinine exclude renal failure. The laboratory findings of normal albumin and trace proteinuria exclude nephrotic syndrome. Most importantly, his physical findings (rales, edema, S_3 gallop) are classic for heart failure.

The relatively low urine sodium (10 mEq/L), high specific gravity (1.024), and high BUN:creatinine ratio suggest that despite an excess of total body sodium, he likely has decreased "effective" blood volume. This coupled with hyponatremia are signs of serious heart failure.

2. Appropriate therapy for heart failure includes salt restriction (and in this patient's case, water restriction, as well). Digitalis, diuretics, and vasodilators all work to increase cardiac output and thus improve "effective" ECV. ACE inhibitors appear to be the vasodilators of choice for heart failure in patients who have normal renal function. They enhance renal sodium and water excretion by their effect on intrarenal hemodynamics (see Table 7-7).

Case 7-4: *Discussion*

1. This case again exemplifies ECV overload (edema) caused by heart failure. Unlike the patient in Case 7-3, however, the severe prerenal azotemia and hyponatremia suggest serious heart failure.

The prerenal azotemia worsened on Day 3 coincident with a 2-kg weight loss and an increase in the amount of diuretics used. In this setting, renal blood flow is severely compromised and relatively "fixed." GFR therefore is increasingly dependent on intrarenal efferent arteriolar constriction due to angiotensin II, raising intraglomerular hydrostatic pressure. ACE inhibitor therapy in such a patient may cause a precipitous drop in GFR as the ES dilates and glomerular hydrostatic pressure decreases. The compensatory increase in renal blood flow required to maintain the GFR is not possible because of the compromised renal blood flow in this overly diuresed patient (see Table 7-7).

2. On Day 5, the diuretics should be withheld. With relatively mild cases, the azotemia may resolve without the ACE inhibitor being discontinued. Low-dose dopamine (1 to 3 µg/kg/min) may improve renal blood flow, improving GFR and azotemia.

3. With severe heart failure (hyponatremia and prerenal azotemia) this situation is sometimes avoidable if diuretics are withheld for 1 to 2 days before ACE inhibitors are initiated. Low-dose dopamine can even be used prophylactically. Administering very small initial doses of ACE inhibitor (e.g., captopril, 6.25 mg every 12 hours) is also prudent.

Case 7-5: *Discussion*

1. In this patient, cirrhosis is the most likely cause of edema. The normal blood pressure, creatinine, and urinary protein exclude the diagnoses of hyperaldosteronism, renal failure, and nephrotic syndrome, respectively. The physical examination (with its findings of icterus and spider angiomata) and abnormal liver function tests confirm the suspicion of liver disease. A history taken from the family revealed substantial long-term alcohol abuse.

2. The physical examination also reveals an excess of total body sodium (ECV expansion). The hyponatremia indicates water overload. This patient therefore needs salt and water restriction, not IV fluids. If IV access is needed, he should have a heparin lock.

3. The appropriate treatment is salt and water restriction. Gentle diuretics can be introduced, generally a combined program of thiazide type and potassium-sparing diuretics. Potent loop diuretics should be avoided. Low-dose dopamine may be helpful in hospitalized patients over the short-term. If the patient is refractory to these measures, a peritoneal-venous (LeVeen) shunt may be considered.

References

Cade R, Wagemaker H, Vogel S, et al. Hepatorenal syndrome: studies of the effect of vascular volume and intraperitoneal pressure on renal and hepatic function. Am J Med 1987; 82:427–438.

Dzau VJ. Renal and circulatory mechanism in congestive heart failure. Kidney Int 1987; 31:1402–1415.

Dzau VJ. Renal effects of angiotensin-converting enzyme inhibition in cardiac failure. Am J Kidney Dis 1987; 10(suppl):74–80.

Norris SH, Buell JC, Kurtzman NA. The pathophysiology of cirrhotic edema: a re-examination of the "underfilling" and "overflow" hypotheses. Seminars in Nephrology 1987; 7:99–105.

Packer M, Lee WH, Medina N, et al. Functional renal insufficiency during long-term therapy with captopril and enalapril in severe chronic heart failure. Ann Intern Med 1987; 106:346–354.

Schrier RW. Pathogenesis of sodium and water retention in high output and low output cardiac failure, nephrotic syndrome, cirrhosis, and pregnancy. N Engl J Med 1988; 319:1065–1072, 1127–1134.

Shapiro MD, Nicholls KM, Groves BM, Schrier RW. Role of glomerular filtration rate in the impaired sodium and water excretion of patients with the nephrotic syndrome. Am J Kidney Dis 1986; 8:81–87.

8 Clinical Disorders of Water Balance:
Hyponatremia and Hypernatremia

- Case Presentations

- Control of Water Balance

- Isolated Disorders of Water Balance (Disorders in Patients with Normal Total Body Sodium)

- Simultaneous Disorders of Water and Total Body Sodium

- Diagnostic and Therapeutic Approach

- Case Discussions

Case 8-1

A 74-year-old woman had peripheral edema, but was otherwise well. Physical examination showed a blood pressure of 140/82 and an absence of rales and jugular venous distention. The cardiac examination was normal. Her weight was 60 kg. She was prescribed chlorthalidone 25 mg daily. Ten days later, she was admitted to the hospital after having fallen. At that time her blood pressure was 124/64 and 90/50 in the supine and sitting positions, respectively, and her pulse rate was 110 beats per minute. She was lethargic and disoriented. The results of the initial laboratory evaluation are shown in the following table.

Na	112	mEq/L
K	2.9	mEq/L
Cl	72	mEq/L
HCO₃	28	mEq/L
BUN	28	mg/L
Creatinine	1.2	mg/dl
Urinary Na	44	mg/dl
Urinary K	40	mEq/L
U$_{osm}$	310	mOsm/L

Questions

1. What is the cause of the hyponatremia?
2. Explain the hypokalemia and metabolic alkalosis.
3. What is the best treatment?
4. If the patient were left untreated, what would the urinary Na and osmolarity be after 24 hours?

Case 8-2

A 79-year-old man was admitted to the hospital for acute left hemiplegia. He weighed 64 kg. His past history was positive for long-standing hypertension and gout. He received IV fluids initially for 2 days. Gradually he became increasingly confused and disoriented. On the 7th hospital day, he had a grand mal seizure. According to the nurses' report he had "excellent" urinary output. Physical examination revealed normal vital signs, normal mucous membranes and an absence of rales, jugular venous distention, and edema. The results of laboratory tests for Days 1 through 9 are shown in the following table.

	Day 1	Day 3	Day 7	Day 9
Na	159.0 mEq/L	146 mEq/L	171.0 mEq/L	148.0 mEq/L
K	4.0 mEq/L	38 mEq/L	39.0 mEq/L	42.0 mEq/L
Cl	105.0 mEq/L	108 mEq/L	124.0 mEq/L	108.0 mEq/L
HCO₃	24.0 mEq/L	26 mEq/L	30.0 mEq/L	25.0 mEq/L
BUN	18.0 mg/dl		29.0 mg/dl	20.0 mg/dl
Creatinine	1.9 mg/dl		2.1 mg/dl	1.8 mg/dl
Urine specific gravity	1.005		1.008	
U$_{osm}$			182.0 mOsm/L	
U$_{NA}$			44.0 mEq/L	

Questions

1. What is the cause of the hypernatremia? How would you confirm your suspicion?
2. What fluids should be administered on Day 7? How much? How quickly?

Case 8-3

A 68-year-old man was admitted to the coronary care unit. He had a long history of hypertension and had been taking hydrochlorothiazide (50 mg daily). For several months before admission, he had had progressive exertional dyspnea and edema. Initial examination revealed blood pressure of 194/112, jugular venous pressure of 10 cm H_2O, bilateral rales, hepatomegaly, probable ascites, and 3+ peripheral edema. Chest radiograph showed bilateral pleural effusion and an enlarged heart. He was to receive routine coronary care and was given furosemide. The results of the laboratory tests for Days 1 through 5 are shown in the following table.

	Day 1	*Day 2*	*Day 5*
Na	126.0 mEq/L	120.0 mEq/L	132.0 mEq/L
K	3.5 mEq/L	3.3 mEq/L	4.2 mEq/L
Cl	90.0 mEq/L	86.0 mEq/L	100.0 mEq/L
HCO_3	26.0 mEq/L	24.0 mEq/L	25.0 mEq/L
Glucose	174.0 mg/dl	142.0 mg/dl	128.0 mg/dl
BUN	26.0 mg/dl	34.0 mg/dl	18.0 mg/dl
Creatinine	1.2 mg/dl	1.3 mg/dl	1.1 mg/dl
U_{NA}		43.0 mEq/L	
U_{osm}		310.0 mOsm/L	

Questions

1. What is the most likely cause of the hyponatremia?
2. What are the factors contributing to the hyponatremia?
3. Why did the hyponatremia worsen on Day 2?
4. What is the appropriate treatment?

Case 8-4

An 86-year-old woman weighing 34 kg was admitted to the hospital after refusing to eat for 2 to 3 days in the nursing home where she resided. Past history was unavailable; however, it was known that she was taking L-thyroxine, digoxin, a stool softener, and aspirin. Physical examination showed a blood pressure of 96/62 and a pulse rate of 128 beats per minute. Neck veins were flat even when the patient was in the supine position. Mucous membranes were dehydrated and the skin possibly "tented." Results of the laboratory tests for the 1st through 48th hour of hospitalization are shown in the following table.

	Admission	12 hrs	24 hrs	48 hrs
Na (mEq/L)	162.0	154.0	152.0	146.0
K (mEq/L)	3.8	2.8	3.5	3.7
Cl (mEq/L)	123.0	125.0	127.0	121.0
HCO₃ (mEq/L)	14.0	16.0	11.0	19.0
Glucose (mg/dl)	135.0			
BUN (mg/dl)	101.0		79.0	60.0
Creatinine (mg/dl)	2.8		1.8	1.4
Ca (mg/dl)	11.6		8.7	8.6
Phosphorus (mg/dl)	3.2		1.1	2.4
U_NA			26.0	
U_cr			50.0	
U_osm			450.0	

Questions

1. What is the cause of the hypernatremia?
2. What is the cause of the azotemia? What would you expect urinary Na and osmolarity to have been on admission?
3. What is the most likely cause of the metabolic acidosis?
4. What treatment should the patient receive on admission?
5. What fluids should be given at 24 hours? How quickly?

Disorders of water balance are reflected by changes in the osmolarity of the extracellular fluid. Osmolarity is the measure of the concentration of osmotically active particles and can be estimated by the formula:

$$\text{Serum osmolarity} = 2([Na] + [K]) + \frac{\text{Glucose}}{18} \text{ (mg/dl)}$$
$$+ \frac{\text{Urea}}{2.8} \text{ (mg/dl)}$$

Normally, the measured serum osmolarity will not exceed this calculated osmolarity by more than 10 mOsm/L. In certain situations, however, exogenous osmoles added to the plasma will increase measured osmolarity, causing it to far exceed this calculated value. Such an "*osmolar gap*" is commonly encountered with intoxication by isopropyl alcohol, ethanol, methanol, and ethylene glycol (the latter two also producing a high anion gap metabolic acidosis) (Table 8-1).

Because serum sodium concentration accounts for almost all osmolarity, it is clinically useful to say that hyponatremia reflects hypo-osmolarity (water excess), whereas hypernatremia reflects hyperosmolarity (water deficiency). However, when very high concentrations of glucose (or mannitol) increase extracellular water, hyponatremia without hypo-osmolarity or hyperosmolarity with a normal serum sodium concentration may result. Because urea is a small molecule and easily permeates all membranes, hyperosmolarity caused by excess urea alone is not clinically significant.

Control of Water Balance

Normally, serum osmolarity is maintained at 280 to 290 mOsm/L by three important mechanisms: thirst, the renal handling of water, and antidiuretic hormone.

Table 8-1 Causes of the Osmolar Gap

Isopropyl alcohol	Ethylene glycol
Ethanol	Hyperlipidemia
Mannitol	Hyperproteinemia
Methanol	

Pseudo hyponatremia – hyperglycemia causes an osmotic shift of H_2O out of cells – for every ↑ of 5 above the Ⓝ b.s (50), the $[Na^+]$ ↓ by 1 meq/L

Because it stimulates water intake, the sensation of thirst is a major defense against hyperosmolarity, maintaining serum osmolarity even in the absence of ADH or renal water conservation. Thirst is stimulated or suppressed by hypothalamic receptors for both osmolarity and effective blood volume (the latter perhaps mediated by angiotensin II). So effective are hyperosmolarity and hypovolemia in stimulating thirst that hypernatremia rarely develops unless the patient has limited access to water.

Figure 8-1 reviews the renal handling of water. Normally water is freely filtered at a rate equal to the glomerular filtration rate (150 L/day). Approximately 80% is isotonically reabsorbed in the proximal tubule. The descending limb of Henle is freely permeable to water but essentially impermeable to solute such that urinary osmo-

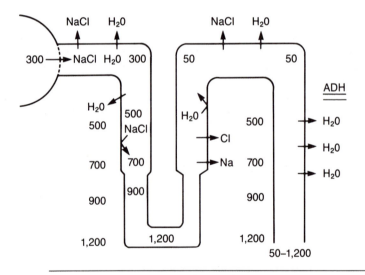

Figure 8-1: Renal handling of water. Numbers represent osmolarity (mOsm/L) of tubular fluid along the nephron. Water is reabsorbed isotonically in the proximal and distal tubules. Urine is diluted (1200→50 mOsm/L) in the ascending limb of Henle (diluting segment) by the active reabsorption of chloride and sodium without water. Urine is concentrated under the influence of ADH in the collecting tubule (concentrating segment).

larity approaches 1,200 mOsm/L in the loop. In the ascending limb, "free water" is created by the active removal of chloride and sodium without water, lowering the urinary osmolarity to almost 50 mOsm/L. The solute removed by the ascending limb is deposited in the medullary interstitium, establishing the medullary concentrations of solute necessary for the eventual concentration of the urine by the reabsorption of water across the collecting tubule. The permeability of the collecting tubule for water is completely dependent on ADH.

The generation and excretion of free water (dilution) is dependent on the ascending limb of Henle (diluting segment), whereas the ability to conserve water (concentration) is dependent on the collecting tubule (concentrating segment). Both processes can be greatly modified by the delivery of tubular fluid to these nephron segments. The delivery of filtrate to these more distal segments is largely determined by the volume of glomerular filtrate and the proximal tubular reabsorption of filtrate. Hence either a decrease in GFR or an increase in proximal tubular reabsorption will significantly limit the ability to dilute or concentrate the urine.

Thus, the four primary factors that determine renal handling of water are (1) GFR, (2) proximal tubular reabsorption, (3) active reabsorption of sodium and chloride in the ascending limb, and (4) water reabsorption in the collecting tubule under the influence of ADH.

ADH release from the hypothalamus is controlled by both osmotic and nonosmotic stimuli (Table 8-2). Of these, serum osmolarity and extracellular volume are the most important. A slight increase in serum osmolarity stimulates ADH release and subsequent renal water reabsorption, restoring serum osmolarity to normal. Similarly, hypo-osmolarity will inhibit ADH release, resulting in a water diuresis. Whereas changes in osmolarity account for the usual, day-to-day control of ADH, large changes in ECV can be more potent and clearly override an osmotic stimulus. Thus, hypovolemic conditions (e.g., excessive gastrointestinal losses of salt) are associated with high circulating levels of ADH, even though the patient may be hyponatremic. Similarly, conditions causing a decrease in the "effective volume" (congestive heart failure, cirrhosis) can appropriately cause high levels of circulating ADH despite hyponatremia.

Table 8-2 Factors That Control (Stimulate or Inhibit) ADH Release

Stimulate	Inhibit
Hyperosmolarity	Hypo-osmolarity
Extracellular volume depletion	Extracellular volume surfeit
Pain	Phenytoin
Emotional stress	Ethanol
Morphine	
Vincristine sulfate	
Cyclophosphamide	
Chlorpropamide	
Clofibrate	
Carbamazepine	

In addition to hyperglycemia, both hyperlipidemia and hypergammaglobulinemia can artifactually lower the serum sodium. These latter two create a test-tube phenomenon only. The total sodium in the blood sample is indexed for a false volume as the lipid or globulin displaces water in the aliquot of serum. Hyperlipidemia and hypergammaglobulinemia affect the serum sodium determination only; they have no effect on osmolarity in vivo.

Isolated Disorders of Water Balance (Disorders in Patients with Normal Total Body Sodium)

The clinician must remember that an alteration of the *serum sodium concentration* indicates a disorder of water balance and bears no relationship to the *total body sodium* (determined by the ECV). Hyponatremia can occur with either an excess of or deficiency in total body sodium or without an alteration of sodium balance at all. A decrease in serum sodium concentration indicates a relative water excess, regardless of total body sodium.

It therefore follows that an assessment of total body sodium is invaluable in the diagnostic approach to the hyponatremic patient.

Once total body sodium has been considered, a rational diagnostic approach to hyponatremia can be constructed (Figs. 8-2 and 8-3).

An absolute excess or deficiency of water in a patient with a normal total body sodium will produce hyponatremia and hypernatremia, respectively. Because there is no abnormality of total body sodium, the physical examination will be normal. Rales,

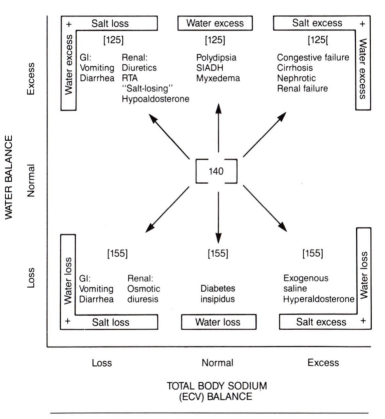

Figure 8-2: Combined water and salt disorders. Water excess (hyponatremia) or deficiency (hypernatremia) can occur with a simultaneous excess or deficiency of total body sodium (ECV).

[Na] < 130 mEq/L

Consider artifact (hyperglycemia, hyperlipidemia, hyperglobulinemia)

Consider ECV

Deficiency — Normal — Excess

	Deficiency: GI loss	Deficiency: Renal loss	Normal: Polydipsia	Normal: Myxedema	Excess
Causes	Vomiting, diarrhea, fistula	Diuretics, RTA, "salt-losing," hypoaldosteronism		Glucocorticoid deficiency SIADH	Congestive failure Cirrhosis/ascites Nephrotic syndrome Renal failure
Findings	U_{osm} of > 450 mOsm/L, U_{Na} of < 10 mEq/L	U_{osm} of 300 ± mOsm/L, U_{Na} of > 30 mEq/L	U_{osm} of 50–100 mOsm/L, U_{Na} of > 30 mEq/L	U_{osm} of > 400 mOsm/L, U_{Na} of > 30 mEq/L	U_{osm} of > 450 mOsm/L, U_{Na} of < 10 mEq/L
Primary Mechanism	Salt loss	Salt loss	Water excess	Water excess	Water excess being greater than salt excess
Secondary Mechanism	Decreased distal delivery	Decreased distal delivery			Decreased distal delivery Increased ADH
Primary Therapy	Saline	Saline	Water restriction	Water restriction	Salt and water restriction
Secondary Therapy			ACE inhibitors	Demeclocycline, lithium, or phenytoin	Digitalis, diuretics, or ACE inhibitors

Table 8-3 Drugs that Cause Hyponatremia

Stimulate ADH	*Increase Sensitivity to ADH*	*Stimulate Thirst*
Chlorpropamide	Chlorpropamide	Thioridine
Clofibrate	Tolbutamide	Thiothixene
Cyclophosphamide	Indomethacin	Amitriptyline
Carbamazepine	Other NSAIDs	hydrochloride
Vincristine sulfate		Fluphenazine
Barbiturates		
Morphine		
Nicotine		

edema, and jugular venous distention will be absent; blood pressure, pulse, mucous membranes, and results of the skin examination will be normal. The only manifestation of the water excess or deficiency will be the altered serum osmolarity (sodium concentration) and its clinical sequela. The syndromes of pure water excess and deficiency and their causes are outlined in Figure 8-2.

Hyponatremia

Hyponatremia that occurs without an alteration in total body sodium is the result of either a massive intake of free water or an inability to excrete water appropriately (i.e., dilute the urine). The normal individual is capable of excreting nearly 20 L of water daily. Nevertheless, there are some patients who can drink nearly that amount every day, overwhelming their renal-diluting capacity. Such patients have "psychogenic polydipsia." (More common, however, are patients who imbibe less water but are taking medications that limit free water excretion, e.g., those listed in Table 8-3). Patients with massive oral or IV intake of water are easily identified by their normal physical examination and by the fact that they dilute urine normally (U_{osm} of 50 to 100 mOsm/L). Because very slight

◄ **Figure 8-3:** Diagnostic and therapeutic approach to hyponatremia.

Table 8-4 Causes of SIADH

Ectopic ADH production
  Carcinomas
  Lymphomas
 	
CNS disorders
  Tumor
  Encephalitis/meningitis
  Abscess
  Head trauma
  Subarachnoid bleed
	Pulmonary disorders
	  Viral or bacterial pneumonia
	  Tuberculosis
	  Lung abscess
	  Positive pressure ventilation

(not clinically detectable) intravascular volume expansion also occurs, the urinary sodium is usually greater than 30 mEq/L. The aim of treatment is to restrict water intake. Captopril has also been used to inhibit AII, a potent dipsogenic substance.

Hypothyroidism, glucocorticoid deficiency, and the syndrome of inappropriate ADH secretion (SIADH) are all associated with inadequate urinary dilution. SIADH has several causes, including malignancies, central nervous system disorders, and primary pulmonary processes (Table 8-4). All are characterized by the continuous, nonsuppressible secretion of ADH, resulting in an inappropriately concentrated urine (usually >400 mOsm/L) despite hypo-osmolarity of serum. Slight (clinically undetectable) expansion of intravascular volume results in a relatively high urine sodium (>30 mEq/L). Mild hypokalemia, hypouricemia, and a low BUN are also commonly seen.

Thus, SIADH occurs in patients with normal total body sodium (without edema), hyponatremia with high urine sodium, hypo-osmolarity with high urine osmolarity, and normal thyroid, adrenal, and renal function (Table 8-5). The aim of treatment is to restrict

Table 8-5 Diagnosis of SIADH

Low serum sodium; high urine sodium (>30 mEq/L)

Low serum osmolarity; high urine osmolarity (> serum osmolarity)

Absence of edema

Normal thyroid, adrenal, and renal function

Correction of hyponatremia with water restriction

free water intake. Further therapy is directed at suppressing ADH secretion (using lithium), interfering with its renal cellular action (using demeclocycline, phenytoin, or lithium), and lowering urinary osmolarity to isotonicity (300 mOsm/L) by the use of loop diuretics.

Hypernatremia

In rare cases, hypernatremia can develop from cutaneous and pulmonary losses of hypotonic fluids (fever and tachypnea with heat-stroke). In general, however, hypernatremia in a patient with a completely normal ECV is caused by renal water loss resulting from diabetes insipidus (DI). Central DI results from a partial or complete lack of ADH secretion usually caused by a central nervous system disorder (Table 8-6). Patients manifest polyuria with an unusually low urinary osmolarity (50 to 100 mOsm/L), an inability to increase urine osmolarity after 8 hours of dehydration, but correction of the defect by ADH administration (aqueous vasopressin, DDAVP). Long-term treatment consists of exogenous ADH.

By contrast, patients with nephrogenic DI have a collecting tubule that is not responsive to ADH. They are not able to increase urinary osmolarity in response to dehydration or exogenous ADH. Treatment is aimed at ECV contraction with diuretics (thiazides

Table 8-6 Etiologies of Diabetes Insipidus

Central DI	Nephrogenic DI
Posthypophysectomy	Congenital DI
Trauma	Interstitial nephritis
Tumors	Multiple myeloma
Craniopharyngioma	Obstructive uropathy
Metastatic	Hypercalcemia
Meningitis/encephalitis	Hypokalemia
Aneurysms	Polycystic DI/medullary cystic DI
Tuberculosis	Sickle cell
Sarcoidosis	Sjögren's syndrome
Histiocytosis	Drugs
Sheehan's syndrome	Lithium
	Methoxyflurane
	Demeclocycline

or amiloride), which stimulates water reabsorption by more proximal nephron segments.

Patients with DI usually do not develop hypernatremia unless they are unable to drink water. The syndrome is therefore usually seen only in patients with a depressed sensorium or an inability to obtain water.

Simultaneous Disorders of Water and Total Body Sodium

Because of the kidney's enormous capacity to conserve and excrete water, the above outlined isolated abnormalities of water balance are relatively uncommon. More likely, salt and water balance are deranged simultaneously such that hyponatremia and hypernatremia are identified in patients with an abnormality of total body sodium. (These abnormalities complete the four quadrants of Figure 8-2.)

Hyponatremia with Low Total Body Sodium (Water Excess with Salt Loss)

Significant gastrointestinal or renal loss of salt will lead to hyponatremia if the patient continues to ingest water. (If the patient is unable to replace water, a normal serum sodium or even hypernatremia can occur with continued insensible loss of water). These patients should demonstrate physical findings of total body sodium depletion, including tachycardia, orthostatic hypotension, dry mucous membranes, and poor skin turgor (see Chapter 7). Although the hyponatremia is caused by salt loss, it is further aggravated by an appropriate hypovolemic stimulus to ADH secretion and decreased delivery of urine to the ascending limb of Henle (diluting segment). This decrease in distal urine flow is caused by increased proximal tubular reabsorption of filtrate (decreased fractional excretion).

This condition occurs with significant gastrointestinal fluid losses from vomiting (usually associated with metabolic alkalosis) or diarrhea (usually associated with metabolic acidosis). In this situation, the kidney appropriately conserves sodium (U_{NA} < 10 mEq/L) and water (U_{osm} > 450 mOsm/L). The aim of treatment is to correct the underlying gastrointestinal disorder while replacing ECV losses with normal saline and potassium.

Hyponatremia caused by renal salt loss is usually caused by the use of diuretics. After therapy has been initiated the hyponatremia should occur within 2 weeks, the time frame of negative sodium balance. It is highly unusual to see hyponatremia as a late complication of diuretic therapy. Metabolic alkalosis and hypokalemia are commonly associated with renal losses of salt. In addition, the severity of the hyponatremia is seemingly related to the degree of hypokalemia.

Other renal causes of negative salt balance include osmotic diuresis (resulting from hyperglycemia or the use of mannitol), mineralocorticoid deficiency, renal tubular acidosis, and rarely, inappropriate renal salt losses caused by tubulointerstitial diseases ("salt-losing nephropathy").

One would expect a high urine sodium (generally > 30 mEq/L) with renal salt-wasting. The urinary osmolarity is generally isotonic (approximately 300 mOsm/L). Treatment consists of discontinuing the diuretic or correcting the underlying disorder when possible. Saline administration will correct volume deficits and hyponatremia.

Hyponatremia with High Total Body Sodium (Salt and Water Excess)

Patients with CHF, cirrhosis with ascites, and nephrotic syndrome are particularly prone to develop hyponatremia despite expansion of total body sodium. In patients with heart failure, ineffective blood volume stimulates ADH secretion and renal water reabsorption from the collecting tubule. Thirst is also stimulated. In addition, the ability to excrete water is limited by a decreased delivery of filtrate to the diluting segment (ascending limb of Henle) caused by decreased renal blood flow and GFR. Diluting capacity may be further compromised by the use of "loop" diuretics (Table 8-7).

Table 8-7 Factors Contributing to Hyponatremia in Patients with Chronic Heart Failure

Increased ADH secretion

Decreased delivery of filtrate to diluting segment
  Decreased GFR
  Increased proximal tubular reabsorption

Loop diuretics

Increased thirst

Intravenous D_5W

D_5W = 5% dextrose in water.

Although the GFR falls in patients with cardiac failure, it does not fall as much as one would expect from a decrement in RBF alone. High circulating levels of AII in patients with CHF cause constriction at efferent arteriolar sphincters, increasing glomerular capillary hydrostatic pressure and blunting the fall in GFR. The fraction of RBF that is filtered (i.e., the filtration fraction) increases, increasing the concentration of plasma proteins in the peritubular capillary. This peritubular rise in oncotic pressure coupled with a decrease in peritubular hydrostatic pressure (caused by ES constriction) enhances proximal tubular reabsorption of filtrate, thus limiting delivery to the loop diluting segment. Thus in patients with CHF, the ability to excrete free water is substantially influenced by AII. (See Chapter 7 for further details on heart failure).

Urinary chemistries usually reflect the intense reabsorption of salt and water caused by the decrease in effective blood volume. Thus, urinary sodium is usually less than 10 mEq/L, FE_{NA} is usually less than 1%, and urine osmolarity is usually greater than 450 mOsm/L (see Fig. 8-3).

Basic therapy for these patients includes restriction of salt and water intake. Digitalis and diuretics may increase cardiac output and effective blood volume. Angiotensin converting enzyme inhibitors (captopril and enalapril) are effective not only as vasodilators, but also for their particular effects on the kidney. By decreasing AII-induced ES constriction, these agents decrease filtration fraction and proximal tubular reabsorption and thus increase delivery of filtrate to the diluting segment. (Figure 8-3 provides diagnostic and therapeutic guidelines for hyponatremic disorders.)

Hypernatremia with Low Total Body Sodium (Salt and Water Loss)

Patients with severe gastrointestinal or renal loss of salt and water are prone to develop hypernatremia, particularly if they are unable to drink water. Severe diarrhea, fistulae, and occasionally, lactulose account for most gastrointestinal causes of this syndrome. Renal salt and water loss is generally associated with an osmotic diuresis such as that caused by hyperglycemia, the use of mannitol, or high-protein (low molecular weight) feedings. Patients with gastrointestinal disorders will appropriately conserve urinary sodium (<10 mEq/L) and water (U_{osm} >450 mOsm/L) whereas patients undergoing an osmotic diuresis will usually have a higher urine sodium (>30 mEq/L) and isosthenuria ($U_{osm} = 300$ mOsm/L) (Fig. 8-4).

In treating these patients, it is best to consider them as having two distinct disorders: a deficiency of total body sodium (ECV) and a deficiency of water (hypernatremia). Despite hypernatremia, one should initially treat severe ECV contraction with isotonic saline, with the volume of saline estimated as a percentage (usually 5 to 15%) of total body water (60% of body weight) (see Chapter 7). When the ECV has stabilized, one can begin to correct the hypernatremia with hypotonic fluid (D_5W). The water deficit can be estimated by the formula:

$$\text{Deficit} = \text{TBW} - \left(\frac{\text{desired [Na]}}{\text{current [Na]}} \times \text{TBW}\right)$$

where

$$\text{TBW} = (0.6 \times \text{body weight [kg]})$$

Hypernatremia should be corrected relatively slowly (over 36 to 48 hours) to avoid the cerebral hemorrhage that results from rapid expansion of the brain tissue.

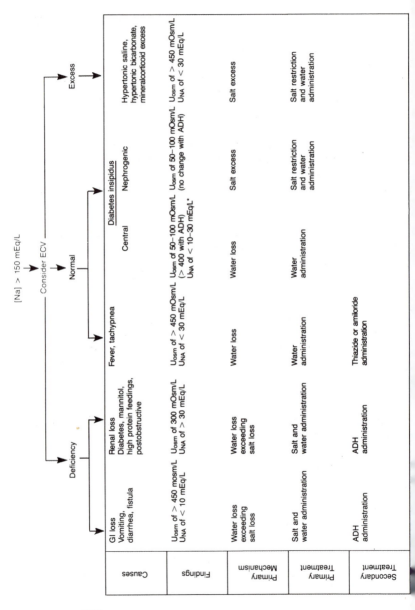

$[Na] > 150$ mEq/L → Consider ECV →

	Deficiency		Normal			Excess
	GI loss	Renal loss	Fever, tachypnea	Diabetes insipidus — Central	Diabetes insipidus — Nephrogenic	
Causes	Vomiting, diarrhea, fistula	Diabetes, mannitol, high protein feedings, postobstructive				Hypertonic saline, hypertonic bicarbonate, mineralocorticoid excess
Findings	U_{osm} of > 450 mosm/L U_{Na} of < 10 mEq/L	U_{osm} of 300 mOsm/L U_{Na} of > 30 mEq/L	U_{osm} of > 450 mOsm/L U_{Na} of < 30 mEq/L	U_{osm} of 50–100 mOsm/L (> 400 with ADH) U_{Na} of < 10–30 mEq/L*	U_{osm} of 50–100 mOsm/L (no change with ADH)	U_{osm} of > 450 mOsm/L U_{Na} of < 30 mEq/L
Primary Mechanism	Water loss exceeding salt loss	Water loss exceeding salt loss	Water loss	Water loss	Salt excess	Salt excess
Primary Treatment	Salt and water administration	Salt and water administration	Water administration	Water administration	Salt restriction and water administration	Salt restriction and water administration
Secondary Treatment	ADH administration	ADH administration	Thiazide or amiloride administration			

230

Hypernatremia with High Total Body Sodium (Salt Excess, Water Loss)

Hypernatremia may develop (albeit rarely) with the acute administration of hypertonic saline (accidental during therapeutic abortion or dialysis) or sodium bicarbonate (administered during resuscitation). Hypernatremia in this setting generally develops acutely and is associated with severe symptomatology. Urinary sodium and osmolarity are both elevated.

Diagnostic and Therapeutic Approach

The diagnostic and therapeutic approach to hyponatremia is outlined in Figure 8-3. In diagnosing hyponatremia, artifacts such as hyperglycemia, hyperlipidemia, and hyperproteinemia are first excluded. Next, one can separate patients according to their total body sodium into those with low, normal, or high ECV. Figure 8-3 lists the common etiologies for each category as well as expected values for urinary osmolarity and sodium. Also listed are basic therapies.

Occasionally, hyponatremia is so severe (<115 mEq/L) or develops so quickly (in less than 24 hours) that symptoms arise and mortality is high. In these patients, rapid correction is desirable. Hypertonic saline (3 to 5%) should be infused at a rate to increase serum sodium by 1 to 2 mEq/L/hr to a serum sodium of 122 to 126 mEq/L. Furosemide can be given simultaneously to avoid extracellular fluid overload.

An approach to patients with hypernatremia is outlined in Figure 8-4. Once again, patients can be separated according to observed changes in total body sodium.

Case 8-1: *Discussion*
1. The physical examination of this patient suggests ECV depletion (tachycardia, orthostatic hypotension). The high urinary

---

◄ **Figure 8-4:** Diagnostic and therapeutic approach to hypernatremia.

sodium, isosthenuria (U_{osm} of 310 mOsm/L), and history of recent diuretic administration suggest that the diuretic is primarily responsible for the hyponatremia.

2. Hypokalemia and metabolic alkalosis are frequently seen in patients who take diuretics. Indeed, the degree of hyponatremia appears to be related to the degree of hypokalemia in these patients. Both hyponatremia and hypokalemia typically develop during the first 2 weeks of therapy.

3. Because of the altered mental status, this patient should receive hypertonic saline (3 to 5%) at a rate to correct the level of her serum sodium to 125 mEq/L over 6 to 12 hours (1 to 2 mEq/L/hr). Thus she should receive 13 mEq/L × 30 L (approximate TBW) or 390 mEq of sodium. This could be provided as 5% saline at 40 ml/hr for 10 hours (500 ml of 5% saline = 425 mEq or approximately 1 mEq/ml).

Failure to correct a patient with symptomatic hyponatremia rapidly may predispose the patient to seizures, respiratory arrest, and permanent brain damage from central pontine myelinolysis and/or postanoxic encephalopathy.

4. Once the effect of the diuretic is gone, the urinary sodium should fall to less than 10 mEq/L and urinary osmolarity should rise to greater than 450 mOsm/L, reflecting a decreased ECV.

Case 8-2: *Discussion*

1. On physical examination, this patient demonstrates a normal ECV. His hypernatremia is therefore the result of water loss. Since he is neither febrile nor tachypneic, renal water loss is the most likely cause. Low urine specific gravity and a U_{osm} of 182 despite hyperosmolarity of the serum confirms this suspicion. The most likely diagnosis is therefore DI.

To differentiate central DI (lack of ADH) from nephrogenic DI (unresponsiveness to ADH) one must observe the U_{osm} response to ADH. When this patient was taking ADH, his U_{osm} increased to only 204, indicating collecting tubule nonresponsiveness to ADH— i.e., nephrogenic DI.

2. Mild ECV depletion and relatively high U_{NA} might also suggest a component of "salt-losing" nephropathy. Both "salt-losing" and nephrogenic DI are commonly seen with tubulointerstitial diseases. Obviously, the water loss (i.e., the DI) was much more severe as the patient developed hypernatremia.

Hypotonic fluids (D₅W) should be administered to this patient. The volume needed to correct the patient to [Na] = 145 mEq/L can be calculated from the following equation:

$$Vol = 38.4 \text{ L} - \left[\frac{145 \text{ mEq/L}}{171 \text{ mEq/L}} \times 38.4 \text{ L}\right] = 5.8 \text{ L}$$

Not more than half of this 5.8 L of D₅W should be administered during the first 24 hours. Administration of hypotonic fluids that is too rapid will cause rapid re-expansion of brain volume, intracranial swelling, and propensity to intracranial hemorrhage.

Case 8-3: *Discussion*

1. This patient obviously has ECV overload. Assuming severe hyperlipidemia and hypergammaglobulinemia to be excluded, his hyponatremia is likely caused by heart failure. (Cirrhosis and nephrotic syndrome must be considered and excluded by examination, chemistry profile, and urinalysis.)

2. Pathophysiologic factors contributing to hyponatremia caused by heart failure include an increased thirst, increased ADH resulting from "ineffective" ECV, and decreased delivery of urinary filtrate to the diluting segment (ascending limb) caused by decreased GFR and increased proximal tubular reabsorption.

3. Most routine coronary orders specify that IV D₅W be administered at variable rates. If hypotonic fluids are administered when the diluting capacity is further compromised by furosemide, hyponatremia will worsen. The U_{NA} and U_{osm} levels on Day 2 suggest that there has been a diuretic effect. Hyponatremia caused by heart failure is associated with low U_{NA} (<10 mEq/L) and high U_{osm} (>450 mOsm/L).

4. Treatment of this patient should be aimed at increasing cardiac output (cardiac inotropes), thus increasing "effective volume" to decrease thirst and ADH and to increase GFR. Diuretic and vasodilator therapy can further improve cardiac output. Distal (metolozone) and proximal (acetazolamide) diuretics should be added if volume overload remains a problem in hyponatremic patients who are receiving loop diuretics (furosemide, bumetanide, ethacrynic acid). ACE inhibitors (captopril, enalapril) are particularly effective vasodilators because they decrease the filtration fraction (GFR/RBF), thus decreasing proximal tubular reabsorption and increasing distal delivery. In addition, intake of salt and water should be restricted. IV medications should be mixed in isotonic fluids (saline) and concentrated to limit the volume infused.

Case 8-4: *Discussion*

1. The hypernatremia indicates a relative water deficiency. The physical examination indicates total body sodium depletion, as well. Because she does not have an obvious history of gastrointestinal fluid loss, this patient most likely lost water (and probably salt) through the kidneys. The hypercalcemia is at least partially responsible for this renal water loss by causing a nephrogenic DI.

2. The azotemia is probably prerenal due to ECV contraction. The relatively low urinary sodium (and calculated FE_{NA} of 0.6%) and high osmolarity at 24 hours support this suspicion. Because the patient had hypercalcemia on admission, one would expect the urine osmolarity at that time to have been much less, probably less than 300 mOsm/L. The urinary sodium would probably have been lower, as well, because of ECV contraction.

3. The metabolic acidosis on admission is of the high anion gap variety, indicating an organic acidosis. Serum salicylate was 2.3 mg/dl and lactate was 1.9 mEq/L, indicating starvation ketoacidosis as the most likely cause of the metabolic acidosis (assuming that the use of methanol, ethylene glycol, and paraldehyde have been excluded). This corrects with hydration (without bicarbonate) due to ketonuria.

4. Because the patient had ECV depletion, isotonic saline should be administered. Five percent depletion would call for approximately 1 L of saline. Administering approximately half of this volume would stabilize the patient enough to permit treatment of the water deficiency (hypernatremia), and D_5W should therefore be administered next. To correct the serum sodium level to 145 mEq/L, one should administer 1.8 L:

$$1.8 \text{ L} = 17 \text{ L} - \left[\frac{145 \text{ mEq/L}}{162 \text{ mEq/L}} \times 17 \text{ L} \right]$$

assuming her TBW is 500% of body weight.

5. Only half of this D_5W should be administered during the first 24 hours so that rapid re-expansion of brain volume and intracranial hemorrhage are avoided.

References

Anderson RJ, Chung HM, Kinga R, Schrier RW. Hyponatremia: a prospective analysis of its epidemiology and the pathogenic role of vasopressin. Ann Int Med 1985; 102:164–168.

Arieff AI. Hyponatremia, convulsions, respiratory arrest, and permanent brain damage after elective surgery in healthy women. N Engl J Med 1986; 314:1529–1535.

Arieff AI. Osmotic failure: physiology and strategies for treatment. Hosp Pract 1988; 23:173–194.

Berl T. Disorders of water metabolism. In: Kurtzman NA, ed. Seminars in Nephrology. Vol. 4. 1984.

Cooke CR, Turin MD, Walker WG. The syndrome of inappropriate antidiuretic hormone secretion (SIADH): pathophysiologic mechanisms in solute and volume regulation. Medicine 1979; 58:240–251.

Dzau VJ, Hollenberg NK. Renal response to captopril in severe heart failure: role of furosemide in natriuresis and reversal of hyponatremia. Ann Int Med 1984; 100:777–782.

Gennari FJ. Serum osmolality: uses and limitations. N Engl J Med 1984; 310:102–105.

Goldman MB, Luchins DJ, Robertson GL. Mechanisms of altered water metabolism in psychotic patients with polydipsia and hyponatremia. N Engl J Med 1988; 318:397–403.

Hantman D, Rossier B, Zohlman R, Schrier R. Rapid correction of hyponatremia in the syndrome of inappropriate secretion of antidiuretic hormone: an alternative treatment to hypertonic saline. Ann Int Med 1973; 78:870–875.

Schrier RW. Pathogenesis of sodium and water retention in high-output and low-output cardiac failure, nephrotic syndrome, cirrhosis, and pregnancy. N Engl J Med 1988; 319:1065–1072, 1127–1134.

9 Clinical Disorders of Potassium Balance

- Case Presentations
- Potassium Homeostasis
- Renal Handling of Potassium
- Causes of Hypokalemia
- Diagnostic Approach to Patients with Hypokalemia
- Causes of Hyperkalemia
- Diagnostic Approach to Patients with Hyperkalemia
- Treatment of Hyperkalemia
- Case Discussions

Case 9-1

A 58-year-old woman was admitted after an apparent syncopal episode. For several years she had been treated for hypertension. Most recently she had been taking triamterene with hydrochlorothiazide (Dyazide) twice daily and clonidine hydrochloride 0.2 mg twice per day with only moderate control of hypertension. Although she had a long-standing complaint of edema, her use of diuretics had been limited because of hypokalemia. Her family history was negative for hypertension.

Physical examination was normal except for a blood pressure of 168/104 and mild peripheral edema. Laboratory examination revealed a normal complete blood count and chemistry profile; serum electrolytes were as follows: sodium, 141 mEq/L; potassium, 2.5 mEq/L; chloride, 98 mEq/L, and HCO₃, 32 mEq/L. The urinalysis was normal. Urine electrolytes were sodium, 43 mEq/L and potassium, 40 mEq/L.

Questions

1. What is the most likely cause of hypokalemia?
2. What diagnostic tests should be performed?

Case 9-2

A 24-year-old woman presented with hypokalemia. Serum electrolytes were as follows: sodium, 137 mEq/L; potassium, 2.4 mEq/L; chloride, 103 mEq/L; and HCO₃, 20 mEq/L. For 6 months she had complained of dizziness and palpitations. She denied vomiting, diarrhea, or other symptoms. She was taking no medications. Past medical history and family history were negative for renal, gastrointestinal, or neurologic disease. Physical examination was normal except for orthostatic hypotension; she had a blood pressure of 112/70 when supine and 88/54 when sitting. Urinalysis was normal, with a pH of 5. The urinary sodium was 8 mEq/L, and the urinary potassium was 16 mEq/L.

Questions

1. What is the most likely cause of her hypokalemia?
2. How would you confirm your suspicion?

Case 9-3

A 19-year-old man was referred for evaluation of hyperkalemia (potassium of 6.7 mEq/L). At one year of age, he underwent right nephrectomy for a Wilms' tumor. At 8 years of age, recurrent Wilms' tumor in the left kidney was treated with segmental resection, chemotherapy, and radiation therapy. He had resultant hypertension and chronic renal insufficiency (creatinine clearance of 28 ml/min) which was relatively stable.

He was taking only atenolol (50 mg daily), furosemide (20 mg twice per day), and hydralazine hydrochloride (50 mg twice per day). He did not smoke, drink alcohol, or use drugs, but he did regularly chew tobacco (Skoal).

His current admission was precipitated by a viral type illness with fever, nausea, diarrhea, and dehydration. He improved with supportive therapy, but his hyperkalemia persisted.

A complete blood count and serum glucose were normal. The results of other laboratory work are shown in the following table.

	Day 1	*Day 4*
Na	136.0 mEq/L	138.0 mEq/L
K	6.4 mEq/L	6.7 mEq/L
Cl	112.0 mEq/L	110.0 mEq/L
HCO_3	18.0 mEq/L	21.0 mEq/L
BUN	88.0 mg/dl	32.0 mg/dl
Creatinine	4.4 mg/dl	2.6 mg/dl
Urinary K		26 mEq/dl

Questions

1. What are the possible factors contributing to his hyperkalemia?
2. What additional tests should be done?

Before discussing the syndromes of hypokalemia and hyperkalemia, we will first review normal potassium homeostasis (Fig. 9-1) and the renal handling of potassium (Fig. 9-2). It is on this normal physiology that our clinical approach to potassium disorders is based.

Potassium Homeostasis

The normal individual ingests approximately 100 mEq of potassium daily. In order to maintain potassium balance, he must excrete 100 mEq daily. Normally, renal excretion of potassium

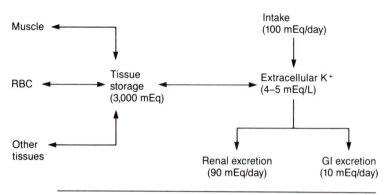

Figure 9-1: Potassium homeostasis.

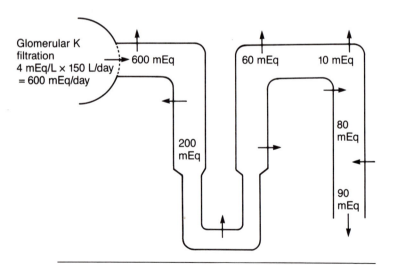

Figure 9-2: Renal handling of potassium. Numbers represent approximate amounts of potassium at different points along the nephron (for all nephrons) per day.

accounts for 90% of daily potassium excretion. However, because the renal capacity for potassium excretion approaches 1,000 mEq daily, hyperkalemia resulting solely from excessive potassium intake is rare indeed.

Most of the total body potassium (>98%) is stored intracellularly in muscle, blood cells, and other tissues. The steep concentration gradient between intracellular potassium (150 mEq/L) and extracellular potassium (4.5 mEq/L) is maintained by a sodium-potassium adenosine triphosphatase (ATPase) dependent pump in the cell membrane and by the integrity of the cell wall. Any shift of potassium from the intracellular to extracellular space may result in hyperkalemia. Alternatively, hypokalemia may arise if potassium shifts intracellularly. The major causes of potassium shift resulting in either hyperkalemia or hypokalemia are listed in Table 9-1.

From this simple schema, one can see that changes in extracellu-

Table 9-1 Causes of Hypokalemia or Hyperkalemia Resulting from Shift of Potassium Between Intracellular and Extracellular Space

Hyperkalemia	*Hypokalemia*
Acidosis (mineral acid)	Alkalosis
Beta₂ blockade	Beta stimulation
Propranolol	Isoproterenol (Isuprel)
Naldolol	Epinephrine
	Albuterol
	Terbutaline sulfate
Alpha stimulation	Alpha blockade
Phenylephrine hydrochloride	Phentolamine
Insulin deficiency	Insulin excess
Hyperosmolarity	Hypo-osmolarity
Aldosterone deficiency	Aldosterone excess
Periodic paralysis	Periodic paralysis
Cell membrane defect	
Rhabdomyolysis	
Hemolysis	
Fluoride intoxication	
Digitalis intoxication	
Succinylcholine chloride	
Mononucleosis	

lar potassium (hyperkalemia or hypokalemia) can result from changes in potassium *intake,* its *shift* across cell membranes, or its *excretion.*

Renal Handling of Potassium

The normal individual filters approximately 600 mEq of potassium daily (4 mEq/L × 150 L/day). For practical purposes, all of the filtered potassium is reabsorbed by the tubules with the proximal tubule reabsorbing 60%, the loop, 30%, and the distal tubule, 10%. Potassium *excretion* is therefore dependent on potassium *secretion* by the distal and collecting tubules. Not only does distal potassium secretion account for all of the 90 mEq normally excreted daily, it also has the capacity to augment potassium excretion in response to excessive intake. The renal handling of potassium is shown in Figure 9-2.

Potassium secretion is directly related to the potassium concentration in the distal tubular cell (Fig. 9-3). Potassium enters the cell via a sodium-potassium ATPase-dependent pump in the peritubular membrane. This pump is strongly affected by aldosterone and pH.

Figure 9-3: Renal potassium secretion is dependent on distal tubular cell potassium (K) concentration. K entry is mostly by an ATPase dependent pump on the peritubular membrane. Acidosis and hypoaldosteronism inhibit this pump. K secretion is enhanced by lumen negativity, exchangeable sodium, and high urine flow rates.

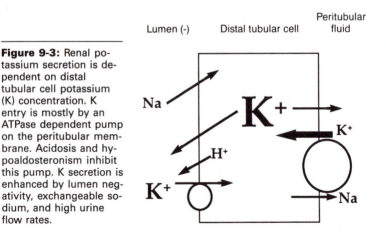

Lumen (-)   Distal tubular cell   Peritubular fluid

Aldosterone and alkalosis promote cellular potassium uptake, whereas hypoaldosteronism and acidosis inhibit uptake.

Once within the cell, potassium diffuses down the electrochemical gradient into the tubular fluid, largely as a result of lumen negativity. The addition of anions to the luminal fluid promotes potassium secretion. This occurs with the accumulation of acetoacetate (during ketosis) and the drug carbenicillin, both of which promote renal potassium wasting.

An increase in the delivery of sodium to distal nephron segments will also enhance potassium secretion. Urine flow has an independent but similar effect. Thus, salt loading and polyuria promote potassium secretion, whereas oliguria inhibits potassium loss. This can be overcome if volume depletion is severe enough to stimulate aldosterone and enhance cellular potassium uptake.

Table 9-2 lists these nonspecific factors which may significantly influence potassium secretion and excretion. Many of these are easily correctable and should therefore be diligently sought and excluded as contributors to either hypokalemia or hyperkalemia.

Table 9-2 Nonspecific Factors Affecting Potassium Secretion

	Promotes Secretion	*Inhibits Secretion*
Na-K ATPase pump	Stimulated Aldosterone Alkalosis	Inhibited Hypoaldosterone Acidosis
Lumen negativity	Nonabsorbable anions Ketones Carbenicillin	
Urine flow/sodium delivery	ECV surfeit Salt loading Polyuria Diuretics	ECV depletion Salt restriction Oliguria
Cell integrity		Tubular/interstitial diseases Potassium-sparing diuretics

Causes of Hypokalemia

Hypokalemia may result from poor intake of potassium, an extracellular to intracellular potassium shift, or excessive potassium-loss (Table 9-3). Poor intake is not a common cause of significant hypokalemia. Cellular potassium uptake is stimulated by alkalosis (ΔK $0.5 = \Delta$ pH 0.1), beta$_2$ stimulation (albuterol, terbutaline sulfate) and insulin therapy, although these rarely cause

Table 9-3 Causes of Hypokalemia

Decreased intake
Redistribution (extracellular to intracellular shift)
    Alkalosis
    Beta$_2$ stimulation (albuterol, terbutaline sulfate)
    Alpha blockade (phentolamine, prazosin hydrochloride?)
    Insulin excess
    Aldosterone excess
    Periodic paralysis

Excessive loss
    Gastrointestinal
        Vomiting/gastric suction
        Diarrhea
        Fistula
    Renal
        Excessive mineralocorticoids
            Primary (Conn's syndrome, Cushing's syndrome)
            Secondary
                Volume contraction (vomiting, Bartter's syndrome, chronic heart failure
                    cirrhosis)
                Renovascular hypertension
                Hypomagnesemia
            Exogenous
                Adrenocorticotropic
                Corticosteroids
                Licorice (Glycyrrhizic acid)
        Nonabsorbable anions
            Na penicillin/carbenicillin
            Ketonuria
        Increased distal sodium delivery
            Diuretics
            Bartter's syndrome
        Renal tubular acidosis

severe hypokalemia. Nearly all cases of serious hypokalemia arise from excessive gastrointestinal or renal potassium wasting.

Hypokalemia commonly accompanies *vomiting* or *nasogastric suction*. However, the concentration of potassium in gastric fluid alone is not high enough to cause the hypokalemia of vomiting (Table 9-4). In fact, in those who vomit, most of the potassium loss is renal. Salt loss and extracellular fluid volume contraction stimulate aldosterone, increasing distal tubular sodium for potassium exchange and renal potassium loss. On the other hand, the concentration of potassium excreted in diarrheal stools may be sufficient to cause hypokalemia. Concomitant hydrochloric acid loss in gastric fluid (causing alkalosis) and bicarbonate loss in diarrhea (causing acidosis) is useful in distinguishing these gastrointestinal causes of hypokalemia (Fig. 9-4).

Renal potassium loss can be a consequence of *excess mineralocorticoid* activity, increased distal delivery of nonabsorbable anions or sodium and renal tubular acidosis. Mineralocorticoids increase distal tubule cellular potassium concentration, which enhances passive diffusion into the lumen. It can be seen with primary aldosterone secretion (e.g., adrenal adenoma), secondary aldosterone secretion (volume contraction, renovascular hypertension or hypomagnesemia), or from an exogenous mineralocorticoid (licorice, Fluorinef). Because mineralocorticoids also increase distal tubular secretion of hydrogen ion, a simultaneous metabolic alkalosis is expected with these disorders.

Nonabsorbable anions may cause hypokalemia. With the exception of chloride and bicarbonate, anions filtered into tubular fluid

Table 9-4 Approximate Sodium and Potassium Concentration in Gastrointestinal Fluids

Gastrointestinal Fluids	Sodium (mEq/L)	Potassium (mEq/L)
Gastric	60–110	10–15
Biliary	140	5
Pancreatic	150	10
Small bowel	80–140	10
Large bowel	120	30

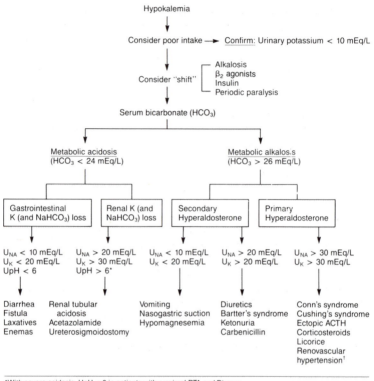

Figure 9-4: Diagnostic approach to hypokalemia.

are poorly absorbed. This increases lumen negativity and potassium secretion. Volume contraction (from renal sodium loss) then stimulates aldosterone, further aggravating hypokalemia and alkalosis. Carbenicillin and ketonuria are common nonabsorbable anions.

Renal potassium loss from *diuretics* (loop and thiazide type) is caused by an increased distal delivery of sodium and urine flow rather than by a direct effect of the drug on potassium secretion per se. Thus, potassium loss caused by diuretics is theoretically limited to the first 7 to 10 days of therapy (the duration of the initial diuresis). The decline in ECV induced by diuretics soon causes compensatory reabsorption of salt and water by proximal nephron segments, thus limiting distal delivery and blunting kaliuresis. If the patient does not simultaneously restrict his salt intake, however, natriuresis and kaliuresis will continue. The patient who develops hypokalemia while taking diuretics should therefore initially receive instruction in dietary salt restriction rather than take potassium supplements. If hypokalemia persists, long-term therapy with potassium chloride is indicated to keep the serum potassium level greater than 3.5 mEq/L.

Bartter's syndrome likely results from a congenital inability to reabsorb sodium and chloride in the loop of Henle. Not surprisingly, this syndrome exactly mimics that caused by diuretic use (i.e., hypokalemic alkalosis with volume contraction and secondary hyperreninemia). Prostaglandin inhibitors and ACE inhibitors have both enjoyed partial success in the treatment of patients with Bartter's syndrome.

Proximal (Type II) and distal (Type I, classical) *renal tubular acidosis* are both associated with severe hypokalemia. The failure to reabsorb bicarbonate in the proximal tubule (proximal RTA) increases distal lumen negativity, distal sodium delivery, and secondary hyperaldosteronism, all of which contribute to kaliuresis. Once again, the kaliuresis is limited by volume contraction. Treatment of these patients with proximal RTA with sodium bicarbonate will only exacerbate the bicarbonaturia and worsen hypokalemia. In distal RTA, potassium secretion is obligated by the inability to secrete hydrogen ion in exchange for sodium. Severe hypokalemia causing respiratory muscle paralysis is often the immediate cause of death in these patients. Treatment with potassium bicarbonate is mandatory for patients with distal RTA.

Diagnostic Approach to Patients with Hypokalemia

A diagnostic approach to hypokalemia based on the above physiology and known differential diagnosis is presented in Figure 9-4. First, poor dietary intake should be considered and confirmed by history and documentation of a low urinary potassium (<10 mEq/L). Next, extracellular to intracellular potassium shifts should be excluded. Severe alkalosis, beta$_2$ agonists, and insulin therapy are the most common causes. Finally, because nearly every cause of potassium loss tends to be accompanied by either metabolic acidosis or alkalosis, the serum bicarbonate concentration provides an easy and efficient differential step in the diagnostic algorithm.

Patients with hypokalemia and metabolic acidosis lose potassium and bicarbonate (usually as $NaHCO_3$) simultaneously in either the gastrointestinal tract or kidney. Gastrointestinal causes include fistula, diarrhea, or laxative and/or enema abuse. If the patient has normal renal function, the urine will reflect renal conservation of sodium ($U_{NA} < 10$ mEq/L) and potassium (urinary potassium < 20 mEq/L) as well as hydrogen ion secretion ($U_{pH} < 6$). If, on the other hand, the kidney is responsible for potassium and (sodium) bicarbonate loss, urinary potassium and sodium will be inappropriately high (urinary potassium > 30 mEq/L, $U_{NA} > 20$ mEq/L) and the urine pH will be alkaline (> 6). This is seen when hypokalemia is caused by RTA or acetazolamide (causing proximal RTA) and with ureterosigmoidostomy.

Hypokalemia with metabolic alkalosis generally indicates a primary or secondary excess of mineralocorticoid. Primary mineralocorticoid excess stimulates potassium secretion for sodium absorption, usually causing ECV overload and hypertension to result. Because of sodium retention, a "mineralocorticoid escape" eventually occurs (see Chapter 7), increasing both urinary sodium and potassium excretion ($U_{NA} > 30$ mEq/L, urinary potassium > 30 mEq/L). With mineralocorticoid activity, adrenal secretion of aldosterone or exogenously administered substances (prednisone, licorice [glycyrrhizic acid]) will also produce this syndrome of fluid retention, hypertension, and hypokalemic alkalosis.

Renovascular hypertension is included in this syndrome of fluid retention, although in reality, renovascular hypertension is a form of secondary hyperaldosteronism. If unilateral renovascular stenosis exists, patients are volume-contracted with renin angiotensin–mediated hypertension. If bilateral stenosis occurs, volume-mediated hypertension with normal plasma renin activity is usual. Both unilateral and bilateral renovascular stenosis are prone to hypokalemic alkalosis.

The remainder of patients with hypokalemic alkalosis have hyperaldosteronism secondary to volume contraction, having lost salt in the urine or intestinal tract. Potassium loss is caused by aldosterone-mediated sodium for potassium exchange (caused by vomiting or nasogastric suction), enhanced distal delivery of sodium (caused by diuretics, Bartter's syndrome), or by an increase in lumen negativity resulting from nonreabsorbable anions (ketonuria, carbenicillin). Intense renal sodium retention ($U_{NA} < 10$ mEq/L) distinguishes patients with vomiting or nasogastric suction from those with renal sodium wasting (diuretics, Bartter's syndrome, nonreabsorbable anions).

Causes of Hyperkalemia

Table 9-5 outlines the common causes of hyperkalemia. In addition to changes in intake, distribution, and excretion of potassium, hyperkalemia may be artifactual or spurious. Artifactual hyperkalemia is usually caused by cellular release of potassium when lysis of platelets or WBCs occurs in a "clot" test-tube (serum). The rise in potassium is usually insignificant until the platelet count exceeds 1 million or the WBC count exceeds 100,000. Simultaneous testing of potassium in a "non-clot" test-tube (plasma potassium) will confirm the phenomenon. Pseudohyperkalemia can also arise after phlebotomy from an ischemic limb.

Unless the renal capacity for excretion of potassium is limited, severe hyperkalemia will not develop from increased intake of potassium alone. Nevertheless, exogenous potassium may often change mild hyperkalemia into a life-threatening problem. Some of the occult sources of exogenous potassium include salt substitutes, stored blood, antibiotics (K penicillin, sterile ticarcillin disodium and clavulanate potassium [Timentin], amoxicillin/clavulanate potassium [Augmentin]), and oral tobacco products.

The causes of intracellular to extracellular potassium shift are listed in Table 9-1. Nonselective beta-blockers, hyperchloremic acidosis, and insulin deficiency are not uncommon causes of mild hyperkalemia. Severe hyperkalemia can result when cell damage or lysis occurs, as with rhabdomyolysis or hemolysis ($\Delta Hgb\ 1\ g = \Delta K^+$ 3.3 mEq/L), particularly when renal excretion is also impaired.

Table 9-5 Causes of Hyperkalemia

Artifact (Pseudohyperkalemia)
  Thrombocytosis (> 1,000,000)
  Leukocytosis (> 100,000)
  Ischemic phlebotomy

Increased intake
  Salt substitutes (50–100% KCl)
  Stored blood
  K penicillin (1.7 mEq/million units)
  Clavulinic acid (0.3 mEq/g of ticarcillin disodium [Timentin])
  Chewing tobacco

Redistribution (intracellular to extracellular shift)

Decreased excretion
  Filtration (GFR ≤5 ml/min)
  Secretion (GFR >5 ml/min)
    Distal cell disease
      Interstitial nephritis
      Renal transplant
      Obstructive uropathy
      Sickle cell disease
      Amyloid
      Other renal parenchymal diseases
    Hypoaldosteronism
      Hyporeninemia
        Diabetes
        Other renal diseases
        Prostaglandin deficiency
        NSAIDs
        Idiopathic hyporeninemia
      AII deficiency
        ACE inhibitors
      Hypoaldosteronism
        Enzyme deficiency
        Addison's disease
        Idiopathic hypoaldosteronism
        Heparin
    Drugs
      Potassium-sparing diuretics
        Spironolactone (Aldactone)
        Triamterene (Dyrenium, Dyazide, Maxide)
        Amiloride (Midamor, Moduretic)
      Cyclosporine
      Digitalis intoxication

Most hyperkalemia results from a defect in distal tubular potassium secretion, which often occurs despite relative preservation of glomerular filtration rate (> 5 ml/min). Because both potassium and hydrogen ion are similarly secreted in exchange for sodium in the distal tubule, secretory potassium defects are usually associated with a hyperchloremic (non-anion gap) metabolic acidosis. Indeed, the association of hyperkalemia with hyperchloremic metabolic acidosis has acquired the term "Type IV" renal tubular acidosis. Loosely included in this category are various causes of renal parenchymal disease (usually with a component of interstitial nephritis) as well as defects in the renin-angiotensin-aldosterone axis producing hypoaldosteronism.

Although the syndrome of "hyporeninemic hypoaldosteronism" may be idiopathic, it is usually (in 70% of cases) associated with various renal diseases, among which diabetes is the most common. Because prostaglandins appear necessary for renin release, most nonsteroidal anti-inflammatory drugs (NSAIDs) are reported to cause or aggravate this hyperkalemic syndrome. Hypoaldosteronism may also occur with normal plasma renin activity producing the same clinical syndrome.

Diagnostic Approach to Patients with Hyperkalemia

When evaluating the hyperkalemic patient (Fig. 9-5), "pseudohyperkalemia" should be excluded and the common causes of redistribution (cellular shift) considered (see Table 9-1). If neither of these appears significant, the urinary potassium can be used to distinguish excessive potassium intake (urinary potassium > 60 mEq/L) from decreased potassium excretion (urinary potassium < 40 mEq/L).

Clinically, a relative excess in potassium intake and mild decrease in renal excretion commonly coexist in the hyperkalemic patient. One should therefore remember the occult sources of exogenous potassium as well as the subclinical causes of defective potassium secretion outlined in Table 9-5. Often, mild to moderate hyperkalemia with mild hyperchloremic acidosis is the only clue to an

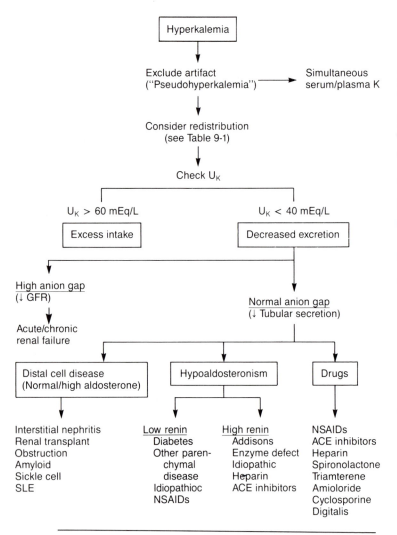

Figure 9-5: Diagnostic approach to hyperkalemia.

underlying hormonal or renal parenchymal disorder ("Type IV" RTA).

Decreased excretion of potassium may result from decreased filtration or secretion. In the case of the former, simultaneous retention of organic acids (phosphates, sulfates) raises the anion gap. Decreased tubular secretion of potassium does not alter the anion gap. Even in those situations where hydrogen ion is also retained, hyperchloremia maintains the anion gap despite metabolic acidosis. Thus, a normal anion gap indicates defective tubular potassium secretion caused by cellular disease, defects in the renin-angiotensin-aldosterone axis, or a drug effect.

A plasma aldosterone level should easily separate those disorders related to hypoaldosteronism (low aldosterone levels) from the group of renal parenchymal diseases that commonly cause decreased potassium secretion (normal or high aldosterone levels). The hypoaldosterone syndromes can be further separated by the plasma renin level into those related to low renin (hyporeninemic hypoaldosteronism) or the reactive hyperreninemic syndromes of adrenal disease, aldosterone inhibitors (heparin), and ACE inhibitors.

More often than not, the cause or causes of hyperkalemia become apparent by simply considering this diagnostic algorithm. Plasma aldosterone and renin levels are usually unnecessary. Nevertheless, these tests may be needed and are often helpful in determining which patients will benefit from mineralocorticoid replacement therapy (Fluorinef).

Treatment of Hyperkalemia

The treatment of hyperkalemia is outlined in Table 9-6. Mild hyperkalemia (less than 5.5 mEq/L) generally requires no specific therapy. However, avoidance of those nonspecific factors precipitating severe hyperkalemia is extremely important (see Table 9-2). Thus, potassium-sparing diuretics, NSAIDs, and ACE inhibitors should be withheld, good urine volume maintained, and dietary potassium restricted.

As serum potassium rises to between 6 and 6.5 mEq/L, peaked T

Table 9-6 Treatment of Hyperkalemia

Serum Potassium (mEq/L)	ECG	Treatment	Onset/Duration	Mechanisms
		Avoid oliguria, K^+ sparing diuretics and NSAIDS		
≤ 5.5	Normal	Restrict dietary K^+		
6	Peaked T wave	Diuretics (Lasix 40–80 IV)	With diuresis	Renal excretion
		Kayexalate (25–50 g PO or PR)	1–2 hours/4–6 hours	GI excretion
7	Prolonged PR Widened QRS	Glucose/insulin (50 g glucose/ 20 Units of regular insulin)	30 min/4–6 hours	Redistribution
		$NaHCO_3$ (50–100 mEq IV)	5–10 min/2 hours	Redistribution
		Albuterol (1 mg inhalation)	30 min/2–4 hours	
8	"Sign wave"	Calcium gluconate (10%; 10–20 ml IV)	1–3 min/0.5–1 hour	Membrane antagonism*

*Calcium increases threshold for depolarization, antagonizing the effect of potassium to increase resting membrane potential.
ECG = electrocardiogram.

waves become apparent on the ECG. Potassium at this level should respond to increased renal or gastrointestinal excretion (promoted by diuretics and sodium polystyrene sulfonate [Kayexalate], respectively). The dose of diuretic may need to be increased (to 80 to 160 mg of IV furosemide) as serum creatinine rises. Kayexalate creates a significant sodium load which may also necessitate an increase in diuretic dose. Oral Kayexalate must be given with a cathartic (20 to 70% sorbitol, 15 to 50 ml) to be effective. Generally, diuretics and Kayexalate must be repeated every 6 to 8 hours.

Higher levels of serum potassium may require more urgent treatment. A shift of potassium intracellularly can be accomplished by sodium bicarbonate, glucose/insulin (ratio usually 2 g/unit), or inhaled albuterol. The duration of this effect is limited, however, so that measures to remove potassium (diuretics, Kayexalate, dialysis) must be undertaken simultaneously.

Life-threatening hyperkalemia may occur at a serum potassium level of 7 mEq/L or greater. This occurs as hyperkalemia increases the resting membrane potential of cardiac cells, blocking depolarization. Calcium increases the depolarization threshold, restoring normal conduction. Again, the effect is very transient and measures for removing potassium must also be instituted.

Case 9-1: *Discussion*

1. Hypokalemia with metabolic alkalosis generally means that there is an excess of mineralocorticoid. This may be primary (e.g., primary hyperaldosteronism) or secondary to ECV depletion. In this patient, physical examination reveals hypertension and edema. Since both are signs of excess ECV, primary hyperaldosteronism (Conn's syndrome) or another form of excess aldosteronism is suggested. The urinary sodium (43 mEq/L) and urinary potassium (40 mEq/L) are supportive of this diagnosis.

2. Confirmatory diagnostic tests should include basal and postdexamethasone serum cortisols to exclude Cushing's syndrome, serum aldosterone levels in the basal state and after saline infusion. In this patient, the cortisol levels were normal but her basal serum aldosterone level was elevated and not suppressed after she received 1 L of saline intravenously. A CT scan of the abdomen (and subsequent adrenalectomy) confirmed the presence of an adrenal adenoma. Subsequently, electrolytes and blood pressure returned to normal.

Case 9-2: *Discussion*

1. Hypokalemia associated with metabolic acidosis means that there has been either gastrointestinal or renal potassium and bicarbonate loss (see Fig. 9-4). Certainly, the gastrointestinal causes of bicarbonate loss (e.g., diarrhea) are far more common than the renal causes (e.g., RTA). Therefore, based on probability alone, diarrhea or laxative abuse would appear to be the cause of hypokalemia and hyperchloremic metabolic acidosis in most patients.

2. The urinary electrolytes and pH easily distinguish this patient as having had diarrhea. Diarrhea causes renal sodium and potassium conservation ($U_{NA} < 10$ mEq/L; $U_K < 20$ mEq/L) and acid excretion (urinary pH < 6) consistent with the values of this patient. On the other hand, RTA causes renal wasting of sodium, potassium and bicarbonate ($U_{NA} > 20$ mEq/L; urinary potassium > 30 mEq/L; urinary pH > 6).

When confronted, the patient admitted to laxative and enema abuse. Often, phenolphthalein present in some laxatives can be detected as a pink color when sodium hydroxide is added to a stool sample.

Case 9-3: *Discussion*

1. In this patient, pseudohyperkalemia is excluded by the normal CBC. Hyperchloremic acidoses can induce a *potassium shift* from cellular stores to the ECV, and this is one factor contributing to the hyperkalemia. However, the severity of the hyperkalemia and its failure to improve on Day 4 despite an improvement in metabolic acidosis suggest additional contributing factors.

The urinary potassium of 26 mEq/L confirms decreased renal excretion of potassium. Since the GFR appears relatively well preserved (> 10 ml/min) and the anion gap is normal, *decreased tubular secretion* of potassium appears likely. Decreased potassium secretion can be caused by tubular cell disease (e.g., interstitial nephritis), hypoaldosteronism (from a variety of causes), and drugs.

2. The patient denied having used other drugs, including nonsteroidal anti-inflammatory drugs. He did have biopsy-proven *interstitial nephritis,* however, and this likely contributed significantly to his hyperkalemia. Other factors causing tubular cell disease (e.g., SLE, sickle cell, amyloid) should also be excluded. Because *hyporeninemic hypoaldosteronism* is commonly associated with hyperkalemia and interstitial nephritis, plasma renin and aldosterone levels should be checked before and after furosemide administration (after other medications are discontinued for 7 days). In this patient, both plasma renin and aldosterone levels were low and did not increase significantly after furosemide-induced volume contraction, confirming hyporeninemic hypoaldosteronism.

One final factor potentially aggravating his hyperkalemia was his regular use of oral tobacco products, a rich "dietary" source of potassium.

References

Cox M, Sterns RH, Singer I. The defense against hyperkalemia: the roles of insulin and aldosterone. N Engl J Med 1979; 300:1087–1089.

DeFronzo RA. Hyperkalemia and hyporeninemic hypoaldosteronism. Kidney Int 1980; 17:118–134.

Fulop M. Serum potassium in lactic acidosis and ketoacidosis. N Engl J Med 1979; 300:1087–1089.

Nardone DA, McDonald WJ, Girard DE. Mechanisms in hypokalemia: clinical correlation. Medicine 1978; 57:435–446.

10 Metabolic Acid-Base Disorders

- Case Presentations

- Metabolic Acidosis

- Renal Tubular Acidosis

- Metabolic Alkalosis

- Mixed Acid-Base Disturbances

- Case Discussions

Case 10-1

A 57-year-old woman was admitted to the hospital with weakness, dyspnea, and an acute state of confusion. A right lower lobe pneumonia was identified on the initial chest x-ray examination (aspiration was suspected clinically).

Medical history included a diagnosis of Sjögren's syndrome made 2 years earlier. This was primarily manifested as keratoconjunctivitis sicca and hypergammaglobulinemia.

Physical examination revealed a blood pressure of 104/60, a pulse rate of 96 beats per minute, and respiration of 36 breaths per minute. Her weight was 60 kg. She was disoriented, and she had a symmetrical decrease in muscular strength $(4+/5+)$. Deep tendon reflexes were absent. The results of the laboratory tests and urinalysis are shown in the following table.

	Laboratory		Urinalysis
Na	140.0 mEq/L	pH	6.5
K	2.3 mEq/L	Na	95.0 mEq/L
Cl	124.0 mEq/L	Cl	92.0 mEq/L
HCO₃	3.0 mEq/L	K	11.0 mEq/L
BUN	25.0 mg/dl		
Creatinine	1.7 mg/dl		
Glucose	99.0 mg/dl		
Calcium	6.7 mg/dl		
Phosphorus	2.1 mg/dl		
pH	7.03		
pCO₂	12.0 mm Hg		
pO₂	96.0 mm Hg		

Questions

1. What is the most likely cause of the metabolic acidosis?
2. What is the most likely etiology?
3. How should the patient be managed acutely? What are the acute complications of therapy?

Case 10-2

A 74-year-old man with chronic obstructive pulmonary disease presented with gross rectal bleeding and abdominal pain. A bleeding adenocarcinoma was found in the descending colon and a left colectomy with colostomy was performed. Postoperatively he had persistent ventilator dependence (for which he received hydro-cortisone sodium succinate [Solu-Cortef]) and ileus requiring naso-gastric suction (as many as 4 L daily). He also had oliguria and azotemia.

His physical examination revealed a blood pressure of 98/60 and pulse rate of 124 beats per minute. His weight was 74 kg. His neck veins were flat despite supine position. There was no edema or rales. The skin tented easily, and the abdomen was markedly distended without bowel sounds.

The results of his laboratory work on the 1st and 5th postoperative days and the results of his urinalysis for the 5th postoperative day are shown in the following table.

| | Laboratory | | Urinalysis |
	Day 1	Day 5	Day 5
Na	140.0 mEq/L	144.0 mEq/L	Na 2 mEq/L
K	4.2 mEq/L	2.6 mEq/L	K 42 mEq/L
Cl	99.0 mEq/L	81.0 mEq/L	Cl 8 mEq/L
HCO$_3$	28.0 mEq/L	48.0 mEq/L	pH 5
pH	7.38	7.70	
pCO$_2$	48.0 mm Hg	40.0 mm Hg	
BUN	22.0 mg/dl	74.0 mg/dl	
Creatinine (mg/dl)	1.5 mg/dl	1.8 mg/dl	

Questions

1. What is the cause of his metabolic alkalosis on admission?
2. What are the acid-base disturbances on Day 5?
3. Why does the urine have a pH of 5?
4. What treatment should be initiated on Day 5?

Case 10-3

A 54-year-old diabetic woman was admitted to the hospital on the 4th day of an acute illness characterized by fever (39.5°C), chills, myalgia, and diarrhea. She denied taking any medications, drugs, or alcohol.

Physical examination showed a blood pressure of 84/52 (in the supine position), a pulse rate of 118 beats per minute, and a labored respiration of 40 breaths per minute. Mucous membranes were dry, neck veins were flat, and there was no edema. The abdomen was distended, firm, and mildly tender but with hyperactive bowel sounds. Her hemoglobin was 15.5 g/dl, hematocrit 48%, WBC count was 22,300 with 66% segmented neutrophils and 23% band forms. Other laboratory values are shown in the following table.

Na	138.0 mEq/L
K	4.2 mEq/L
Cl	108.0 mEq/L
HCO₃	10.0 mEq/L
BUN	38.0 mg/dl
Creatinine	2.4 mg/dl
Glucose	343.0 mg/dl
Ketones	None
Lactate	3.0 mEq/L
pH	7.39
pCO₂	17.0 mm Hg

Questions

1. What is the acid-base disturbance?
2. What is the most likely cause of the metabolic acidosis?
3. What additional laboratory tests should be ordered?

In body fluids, the hydrogen ion concentration, $[H^+]$, or pH is determined by the relationship of two variables, carbon dioxide partial pressure (pCO_2) and bicarbonate (HCO_3). This relationship is best expressed by the Henderson equation:

$$[H^+] = 24 \times \frac{pCO_2}{HCO_3}$$

where 24 is a constant.

The Henderson equation can easily be used clinically by remembering seven numbers—i.e., the $[H^+]$ at any given pH (Table 10-1). Because respiration controls pCO_2 and the kidneys control HCO_3, this expression defines the spectrum of respiratory (changes in pCO_2) and metabolic (changes in HCO_3) acid-base disorders. Acidosis and alkalosis refer to changes in either serum HCO_3 or pCO_2; acidemia and alkalemia refer to changes in pH.

Table 10-2 outlines the primary (initiating) acid-base disturbances and their secondary compensatory changes. Metabolic acidosis is a primary decrement in serum HCO_3 (<24 mEq/L) which results in a decreased pH (acidemia). Secondary stimulation of the

Table 10-1 Relation of Hydrogen Ion Concentration [H⁺] to pH

$[H^+]$	pH
7.60	24
7.50	30
7.40	40
7.30	50
7.20	60
7.10	80
7.00	100

respiratory center lowers pCO_2 (to <40 mm Hg) through ventilation, thus blunting the effect on pH. Metabolic alkalosis is an increase in serum HCO_3 (to >26 mEq/L), which induces hypoventilation and pCO_2 retention. Respiratory acidosis and alkalosis can be primary disturbances as well, increasing or decreasing pCO_2. Respiratory acidosis causes compensatory renal HCO_3 retention; respiratory alkalosis causes renal HCO_3 wasting.

The appropriate magnitude of the secondary compensation is also shown in Table 10-2. For example, a metabolic acidosis that decreases the serum HCO_3 from 25 to 14 mEq/L should stimulate ventilation, lowering the pCO_2 to 29 mm Hg ($pCO_2 = 1.5(14) + 8$). A primary metabolic alkalosis increasing serum HCO_3 to 45 mEq/L should decrease ventilation physiologically to allow a pCO_2 of 52

Table 10-2 The Primary Acid-Base Disturbances With Qualitative and Quantitative Compensation

Primary Disorder		Secondary Compensation	
Metabolic acidosis	$\downarrow HCO_3^-$	$\downarrow PCO_2$	$\Delta pCO_2 = 1.2\Delta HCO_3^-$ or $pCO_2 = HCO_3^- (1.5) + 8$
Metabolic alkalosis	$\uparrow HCO_3^-$	$\uparrow pCO_2$	$\Delta pCO_2\ 6 = \Delta HCO_3^-\ 10$
Respiratory acidosis	$\uparrow pCO_2$	$\uparrow HCO_3^-$	Acute: $\Delta HCO_3^-\ 1 = \Delta pCO_2\ 10$ Chronic: $\Delta HCO_3^-\ 3.5 = \Delta pCO_2\ 10$
Respiratory alkalosis	$\downarrow pCO_2$	$\downarrow HCO_3^-$	Acute: $\Delta HCO_3^-\ 2 = \Delta pCO_2\ 10$ Chronic: $\Delta HCO_3^-\ 5 = \Delta pCO_2\ 10$

Table 10-3 Causes of Respiratory Acidosis and Alkalosis

Alkalosis (increased ventilation)	Acidosis (decreased ventilation)
Central nervous system disease	Central nervous system disease
Hypoxia	Neuromuscular disease
Hepatic failure	Obstructive airway diseases
Salicylates	Mechanical chest wall or pulmonary
Sepsis	disease

mm Hg ($\Delta pCO_2\ 6 = \Delta HCO_3\ 10$). Similar definitions of appropriate secondary compensation are listed for respiratory acidosis and alkalosis. Thus, the compensatory changes serve to dampen the change in pH induced by the primary disturbance, causing the pH to return (although never completely) towards normal.

Any significant quantitative deviation from the listed formula for a compensatory change suggests a second primary disorder or *"mixed" acid-base disorder.* In the above metabolic acidosis example, with the HCO_3 decreasing to 14 mEq/L, a pCO_2 of 24 mm Hg would indicate "overcompensation," which in reality is the presence of a second primary disorder—i.e., respiratory alkalosis. This is true despite acidemia (pH 7.39 = 41 = 24(24 ÷ 14)). It is therefore important that the astute clinician know these formulae defining appropriate compensatory changes so that a second primary disorder (and its differential diagnosis) are not missed.

The general causes for primary respiratory acidosis and alkalosis are listed in Table 10-3.

Metabolic Acidosis

The anion gap (AG), calculated by subtracting the commonly measured anions (chloride [Cl^-] and bicarbonate [HCO_3^-]) from the commonly measured cation (Na^+), serves as a guide to classifying metabolic acidosis. Normally, the AG is 12 ± 2. In reality of course, here is no "gap;" other cations (e.g., K^+, Ca^{++}, Mg^{++}, globulins) and other anions (e.g., PO_4^{--}, SO_4^{--}, albumin) equally balance the positive and negative charges in solution. Nevertheless, because these "other" cations and anions remain relatively static, the difference between the (Na^+) and ($Cl^- + HCO_3^-$)

conveniently divides metabolic acidosis into two distinct groups: those disorders causing the accumulation of acid as hydrochloric acid (HCl⁻) (hyperchloremic acidosis) and those accumulating non-chloride acid (organic acidosis).

Figure 10-1 demonstrates the utility of the AG in three patients.

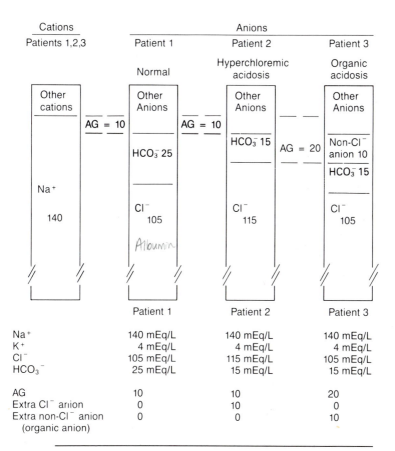

	Patient 1	Patient 2	Patient 3
Na⁺	140 mEq/L	140 mEq/L	140 mEq/L
K⁺	4 mEq/L	4 mEq/L	4 mEq/L
Cl⁻	105 mEq/L	115 mEq/L	105 mEq/L
HCO₃⁻	25 mEq/L	15 mEq/L	15 mEq/L
AG	10	10	20
Extra Cl⁻ anion	0	10	0
Extra non-Cl⁻ anion (organic anion)	0	0	10

Figure 10-1: The utility of the AG in identifying patients with hyperchloremic acidosis and organic acidosis.

✱ for every ↓10 below Albumin of 40 the expected Ⓝ anion gap is ↓ 3 or 4

Patient 1 has normal electrolytes, a normal AG, and no acidosis. In Patient 2, HCl has been added to the system. Each mEq of H^+ which titrates an mEq of HCO_3 is accompanied by a mEq of Cl^-. The decrease in serum HCO_3 to 15 mEq/L is thus offset by a rise in serum Cl^- (hyperchloremic acidosis) and the AG does not change. In Patient 3, the H^+ added to the system is accompanied by a non-Cl^- or organic anion (e.g., H^+ lactate). Therefore, no change in serum Cl^- will occur as the HCO_3 decreases to 15 mEq/L. Rather, a non-Cl^- anion (in this case, lactate) accumulates which should be measured. The AG, however, will increase to 20, identifying this accumulation of non-Cl^- anions as organic acidosis.

Organic Acidosis

The types and causes of *organic acidoses* are listed with their offending acids in parentheses (Table 4). Starvation keto-acidosis is usually mild and easily reversible by dextrose solution. Alcoholic and diabetic ketoacidosis can both be quite severe. Alcoholic ketosis is often associated with high concentrations of beta hydroxybutyrate which does not react to routine ketone-testing and therefore requires specific assay to determine. Lactic acidosis usually results from tissue hypoxia due to hypotension, severe hypoxemia, sepsis or profound anemia. Occasionally, however, significant degrees of lactic acidosis can develop from hepatic failure, seizures, or malignancy, with acidosis caused by the latter being particularly difficult to treat. Uremic acidosis rarely raises the AG to more than 20; higher values indicate an additional organic acid. Both methanol and ethylene glycol will raise the osmolar gap as well as the AG. The simultaneous occurrence of high AG metabolic and a primary respiratory alkalosis suggests salicylate intoxication.

With a pure organic acid acidosis (high AG) the change in serum HCO_3 should approximate the change in the AG. Thus, a lactic acidosis which decreases serum HCO_3 by 10 mEq/L should raise the AG by 10 (i.e., $\Delta HCO_3 = \Delta AG$). A change in AG greater than the lactate level suggests that the presence of additional organic acids such as PO_4^{--} and SO_4^{--} in uremia or acetoacetate in keto-acidosis. If the decrease in serum HCO_3 is greater than the ΔAG, a combined organic and hyperchloremic acidosis is likely. Therefore

Table 10-4 Common Etiologies of Metabolic Acidosis With the Offending Organic Acid in Parentheses

Hyperchloremic Acidoses (AG 12+ or −2)*	Organic Acidoses (AG >14)
Hypokalemic (K usually <3.5 mEq/L)	Ketoacidosis (βOH butyrate, acetoacetate)
Proximal (II) RTA	Alcoholic
Distal (I) RTA	Diabetic
Ureteral diversion	Starvation
Hyperalimentation	Lactic acidosis (Lactate)
Acetazolamide	Tissue hypoxia
Hyperkalemic (K$^+$ usually >4.5 mEq/L)	Shock
Hypoaldosteronism	Sepsis
Addison's	Anemia
Hyporeninemic	Hepatic failure
Idiopathic	Seizures
ACE inhibitors	Malignancy
Drugs	Drugs
NH$_4$Cl	Phenformin
NSAIDs	Cyanide
K$^+$-sparing diuretics	Carbon monoxide
Interstitial nephritis	Uremic acidosis (PO$_4^{--}$, SO$_4^{--}$)
Lead nephropathy	Toxins
SLE	Methanol (formic acid)
Sickle cell	Ethylene glycol (oxalic acid/glycolate)
Obstructive uropathy	Salicylate (unknown)
Transplant rejection	
Others	

*Hyperchloremic acidoses usually cause hypokalemia or hyperkalemia.
AG = anion gap.
Parentheses indicate offending organic acid.

If $\Delta HCO_3 = \Delta AG$, organic acidosis should be confirmed with serum assay. The measured organic acid should equal the ΔAG.

If ΔAG is greater than organic acid (mEq/L), one should search for an additional organic acid.

If ΔAG is less than ΔHCO_3, one should search for a simultaneous hyperchloremic acidosis.

Hyperchloremic Acidosis

Table 10-4 classifies the various causes of metabolic acidosis according to the AG. The *hyperchloremic acidosis* (AG of 12 ± 2) can be divided into further classifications based on the level of serum potassium present. With proximal (Type II) and distal (Type I) renal tubular acidosis, potassium is lost in a HCO_3-rich urine. The same is true with urinary diversion to a surgically mobilized bowel loop, particularly an ureterosigmoidostomy. The administration of amino (hydrochloric) acids with glucose (hyperalimentation) tends to cause *hypokalemia* by stimulating intracellular movement of potassium. On the other hand, with hypoaldosteronism, several drugs, and various forms of interstitial nephritis, failure of the renal tubules to secrete potassium or hydrogen ion effectively leads to a *hyperkalemic* hyperchloremic metabolic acidosis sometimes termed "Type IV RTA."

Treatment

The primary treatment for any metabolic acidosis is to treat the precipitating cause. Thus alcoholic and starvation ketoacidosis are treated with dextrose, diabetic ketoacidosis with insulin, and all three with high fluid intake. IV fluids are also aggressively administered to the patient with lactic acidosis while an attempt is made to correct the underlying tissue hypoxia. Uremic acidosis and methanol, ethylene glycol, and salicylate intoxication often necessitate dialysis when severe.

The use of bicarbonate in the treatment of organic acidosis is controversial. Because ketoacids are often excreted in the urine and ketoacids and lactate are converted to HCO_3 in the liver, the use of IV bicarbonate seems unnecessary in the well-hydrated patient. In addition, overly vigorous use of bicarbonate can lead to "overshoot" alkalosis and cause sodium overload. Nevertheless, with severe acidosis ($HCO_3 < 8$ mEq/L) or when hyperventilation fails to keep the pH above 7.20, the judicious use of bicarbonate at intervals to increase serum HCO_3 by 2 to 4 mEq/L seems reasonable. The amount needed in any patient is easily calculated based on HCO_3 distribution in total body water. For example, to raise the serum HCO_3 from 6 to 8 mEq/L in a 70-kg man, one should use the following equation: 2 mEq/L $\times$ 42 L = 84 mEq HCO_3.

Diagnostic Approach

The diagnostic approach to metabolic acidosis is outlined in Figure 10-2. First, one should consider the possibility of a mixed acid-base disturbance by making sure the pCO_2 is appropriately reduced (1.5 $[HCO_3] + 8$). Next, the AG allows easy classification of the metabolic acidosis as hyperchloremic acidosis (AG = 12 $\pm$ 2), pure organic acid acidosis (AG > 14; ΔAG = ΔHCO_3), or a mixed hyperchloremic/organic acidosis (ΔAG > 14; ΔHCO_3 > ΔAG). The hyperchloremic acidosis can be further divided into hypokalemic (K^+ generally <3.5) and hyperkalemic (K^+ generally > 4.5) varieties. Finally, levels of organic acids (e.g., lactate, ketones, salicylate) should be measured to confirm whether single or multiple factors are responsible for the high AG.

Renal Tubular Acidosis

RTA can be easily approached clinically by understanding the physiologic control of renal acid excretion. Figure 10-3 shows the components of acid secretion and excretion by proximal and distal nephron segments. Tables 10-5 and 10-6 list the key physiologic and clinical features of RTA.

Proximal (Type II) RTA

Filtered bicarbonate (HCO_3) is reclaimed and returned to the blood largely by proximal nephron segments (HCO_3 reclamation). To accomplish this, hydrogen ion (H^+) is secreted (tied to sodium [Na^+] reabsorption) and titrates the filtered HCO_3. The

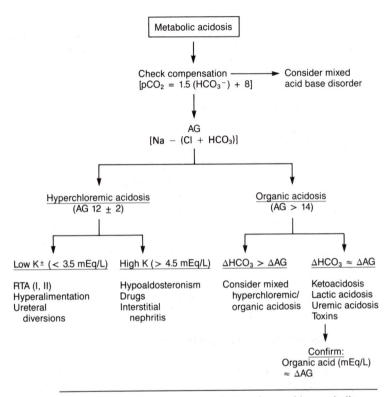

Figure 10-2: Diagnostic approach to patients with metabolic acidosis.

carbonic acid (H_2CO_3) formed rapidly dissociates into carbon dioxide (CO_2) and water by the presence of carbonic anhydrase in the tubular lumen. Cellular carbonic anhydrase allows the cellular resynthesis and subsequent return to peritubular blood of HCO_3. This process reclaims the approximate 3,750 mEq of HCO_3 filtered daily without a change in the luminal pH.

Certain diseases or conditions (Table 10-7) may limit proximal H^+ secretion and thus proximal HCO_3 reclamation, leading to the

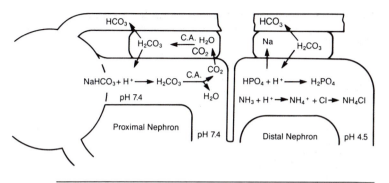

Figure 10-3: The proximal (bicarbonate reclamation) and distal (bicarbonate regeneration) components of renal acid excretion.

clinical syndrome of *proximal RTA*. The resultant bicarbonaturia causes a hyperchloremic metabolic acidosis with inappropriately alkaline urine. Concomitant natriuresis and kaliuresis results in contraction of the extracellular fluid volume and hypokalemia. Since H^+ secretion is usually only partially affected, bicarbonaturia will cease whenever the filtered HCO_3 load falls below the level at

Table 10-5 Clinical Features of RTA

Proximal RTA (disordered reclamation)*	Distal RTA (disordered regeneration)†
Defect in H^+ secretion causing: Sodium bicarbonaturia Hyperchloremic metabolic acidosis High (>6) urine pH Contracted ECV Hypokalemia	Defect in H^+ secretion causing: Hyperchloremic metabolic acidosis Cellular (bone) H^+ buffering Hypercalciuria/hyperphosphaturia Nephrolithiasis/calcinosis Natriuresis/contracted ECV Kaliuresis/hypokalemia
Acid-base balance (and low urine pH) at new steady state of metabolic acidosis	Always positive H^+ balance (urine pH >6)
Treatment: Hydrochlorothiazide and KCl	Treatment: K^+, HCO_3

*See proximal nephron segment of Figure 10-3.
†See distal nephron segment of Figure 10-3.

Table 10-6 Physiologic Control of Acid Excretion

Bicarbonate reclamation*
  Filtered HCO_3 = 3,750 mEq/day (potential loss)
  H^+ secretion/Na^+ reabsorption
  Cellular and luminal carbonic anhydrase
  Reclaimed HCO_3^- (3,750 mEq) with no change in pH
  Largely proximal

Bicarbonate regeneration†
  Endogenous H^+ (1 mEq/kg/day) consumes HCO_3
  H^+ secretion/Na^+ reabsorption
  Cellular carbonic anhydrase only
  H^+ titrated by HPO_4 and NH_3
  pH 4.5 is rate-limiting
  Regenerated HCO_3 = 70 (L/kg) mEq/day
  Largely distal

*See proximal nephron segment of Figure 10-3.
†See distal nephron segment of Figure 10-3.

which the proximal tubule has the capacity to reclaim HCO_3, usually at serum $HCO_3 < 14$ mEq/L. At that point, the patient will be able to acidify urine appropriately (as there is no distal tubular disease) and will be in acid-base balance, albeit at a lower-than-normal serum HCO_3. Administering HCO_3 to these patients will increase the filtered HCO_3, again causing bicarbonaturia and hypo-

Table 10-7 Common Causes of RTA

Proximal (Type II)	Distal (Type I)
Primary (idiopathic)	Primary (idiopathic)
Outdated tetracycline	Dysgammaglobulinemia
Lead	Primary biliary cirrhosis
Amyloidosis	Chronic active hepatitis
Sjögren's syndrome	Sjögren's syndrome
Medullary cystic disease	Medullary sponge kidney
Renal transplantation	Renal transplantation
Multiple myeloma	Nephrocalcinosis
Acetazolamide	Amphotericin B
	Toluene

kalemia. The treatment for patients with proximal RTA is therefore to withhold HCO_3, administer potassium chloride, and induce mild volume contraction with thiazides (or a comparable diuretic). Thiazides nonspecifically enhance proximal tubular reabsorption of sodium, facilitating H^+ secretion and thus HCO_3 reclamation.

Distal RTA (Type I)

In addition to HCO_3 reclamation, the kidney secretes the 70 mEq (1 mEq/kg) of H^+ resulting daily from dietary acid intake and metabolic processes. Tubular H^+ secretion and the cellular presence of carbonic anhydrase thus allows the return to blood or regeneration of the 70 mEq of HCO_3 consumed by endogenous acid production. Because H^+ secretion is limited by a lumen:cell concentration gradient of 1000:1 (at a luminal pH of 4.5) and because less than 1 mEq of free H^+ in the lumen exceeds that gradient, the secretion of 70 mEq of H^+ can be accomplished only by the luminal buffering of H^+ by filtered phosphate (titratable acid) and ammonia synthesized by renal tubular cells. This process of HCO_3 regeneration is accomplished in distal nephron segments.

Impaired distal tubular H^+ secretion and thus HCO_3 regeneration causes the clinical syndrome of distal RTA (see Table 10-5). In these patients, acid accumulates daily, exhausting bicarbonate and other serum buffers. Eventual cellular (bone) buffering results in hypercalciuria, nephrolithiasis and nephrocalcinosis, complications not noted with proximal RTA. Profound hypokalemia results from increased distal tubular Na^+ for K^+ exchange and is often a cause of death. Because patients with distal RTA are unable to secrete H^+ distally, their urine pH remains high despite severe acidemia, distinguishing these patients from proximal RTA. Bicarbonate is mandatory therapy, usually as potassium bicarbonate and citrate (K-Lyte) for patients with distal RTA.

A mixed type of RTA (Type III) with elements of proximal bicarbonate-wasting and impaired distal H^+ secretion is also recognized.

Metabolic Alkalosis

Metabolic alkalosis is a primary increase in serum HCO_3 generated by net alkali gain or net acid loss. The appropriate respiratory response is hypoventilation and pCO_2 retention, the magnitude of which is defined by the formula in Table 10-2, ΔpCO_2 6 = ΔHCO_3 10 (e.g., if serum HCO_3 increases from 25 to 35 mEq/L, pCO_2 increases by 6 to 46 mm Hg).

The normal kidney has a tremendous capability to excrete excess bicarbonate, as bicarbonate reabsorption (reclamation) normally stops at serum levels greater than 28 mEq/L (Fig. 10-4). Thus, once a metabolic alkalosis has been generated, it can be maintained only by the kidney's failure to excrete the excess bicarbonate. This is usually the result of the simultaneous occurrence of hypokalemia (which increases distal Na^+ for H^+ exchange), ECV contraction (stimulating proximal Na^+ for H^+ exchange and HCO_3 reclamation), or hyperaldosteronism (enhancing distal Na absorption and loss of K^+ and H^+). All of these factors increase the bicarbonate reabsorptive capacity, increasing the amount of bicarbonate undergoing reclamation despite the increase in serum HCO_3 and filtered load. Unless these "maintenance" factors are identified and corrected, the metabolic alkalosis will not completely resolve. The

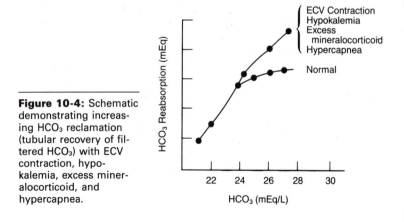

Figure 10-4: Schematic demonstrating increasing HCO_3 reclamation (tubular recovery of filtered HCO_3) with ECV contraction, hypokalemia, excess mineralocorticoid, and hypercapnea.

Table 10-8 Factors Causing the Generation or Maintenance of Metabolic Alkalosis

Generation	Maintenance (failure to excrete HCO_3)
Gain of alkali (HCO_3 or precursor)	Alkali administration
Loss of acid (renal or gastrointestinal)	ECV contraction
	Hypokalemia
	Mineralocorticoid

factors involved in the generation and maintenance of metabolic alkalosis are outlined in Table 10-8.

Table 10-9 classifies the causes of metabolic alkalosis based on the primary factor responsible for their maintenance (continued alkali administration, ECV depletion, hypokalemia or mineralocorticoid excess). Alkali can be administered not only as HCO_3 but also as a precursor (lactate, acetate, citrate) metabolized to HCO_3 in the liver. Hypercapnea causes an endogenous source of HCO_3 by stimulating renal reabsorption. Loss of gastric acid volume generates an alkalosis maintained by ECV contraction. Similarly, diuretics and carbenicillin increase renal acid loss and ECV contraction. All of these causes of metabolic alkalosis are characterized by a very low urinary chloride and are responsive to administered saline, in which case the metabolic alkalosis is "saline-responsive."

Metabolic alkalosis maintained by hypokalemia or excess mineralocorticoid, on the other hand, is "saline-resistant." Causes include Bartter's syndrome, a rare congenital disorder characterized by hypokalemic alkalosis, ECV contraction, and normotension probably arising from defective Na^+ and Cl^- reabsorption in the loop of Henle. Not surprisingly, it is clinically indistinguishable from diuretic abuse. Excess mineralocorticoid syndromes usually cause mild alkalosis with hypokalemia, ECV overload, and hypertension. The "mineralocorticoid escape" phenomenon usually limits the degree of alkalosis and ECV expansion (see also Chapter 7).

The saline-responsive alkalosis (ECV-contracted, hypochloremic) can easily be distinguished from the saline-resistant alkalosis (ECV-expanded, hypokalemic) by the urinary chloride. Because continued urinary loss of sodium and HCO_3 can occur in metabolic alkalosis, the urinary chloride and fractional excretion of chloride

Table 10-9 Etiologies of Metabolic Alkalosis and Primary Factors Responsible for Maintaining the Alkalosis

Etiology	Primary Maintenance Factor

Saline-responsive
  Gastric suction/vomiting
  Chloride diarrhea
  Diuretics
  Nonabsorbable anion
	ECV Contraction

Alkali HCO₃ (exogenous or hypercapnea), lactate, citrate, acetate, antacids	Continued alkali

Saline-resistant
  Primary hyper-aldosteronism
  Adrenal adenoma
  Cushing's disease
  Hyperreninemia
  Liddle's syndrome
  Exogenous mineralo-corticoid
  Licorice
  Use of chewing tobacco
  Prednisone
  Carbenoxolone
	Excess mineralocorticoid

Bartter's syndrome Severe hypokalemia	Hypokalemia

(FE_{Cl}) are superior to urinary Na^+ in confirming ECV contraction. A urine chloride of less than 10 mEq/L (or < 10 mEq/day) indicates significant ECV contraction and saline-responsiveness.

Diagnostic Approach

Figure 10-5 outlines a diagnostic and therapeutic approach to metabolic alkalosis based on the use of urinary Cl^- as an indicator

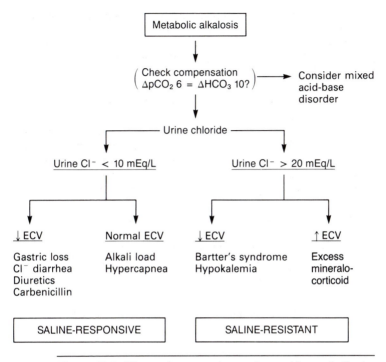

Figure 10-5: Diagnostic approach to patients with metabolic alkalosis.

of saline-responsiveness. First, appropriate respiratory compensation should be confirmed, any significant deviation implicating a mixed acid-base disorder. Next, the urinary Cl^- distinguishes saline-responsive patients (urine $Cl^- < 10$ mEq/L) from saline-resistant patients (urine $Cl^- > 20$ mEq/L). In the group with low urine Cl^-, ECV depletion identifies patients with gastric losses (those caused by vomiting, nasogastric suction) or renal losses of acid and saline (those caused by diuretics, carbenicillin) from those who have gained alkali with normal ECV. In the patients with urinary Cl^- loss (>20 mEq/L), ECV depletion distinguishes those with Bartter's syndrome and severe hypokalemia from those with ECV-expanded mineralocorticoid excess states. Stopping acid loss or alkali gain and administering isotonic saline (usually with KCl) corrects the saline-responsive alkalosis. Saline-resistant patients require vigorous K^+ replacement and a decrease of the mineralocorticoid effect.

Mixed Acid-Base Disturbances

Two or more primary acid-base disorders often occur in the same patient. The pH, pCO_2, and HCO_3 in these situations depend on the relative severity of the disorders and whether they compete or "complement" one another (in a negative sense). The common mixed disorders and clinical examples of each are outlined in Table 10-10.

The clues to a mixed acid-base disorder are

1. Under- or overcompensation of a primary disturbance.
2. Failure to balance compensation formula (see Table 10-2).
3. ΔAG does not equal ΔHCO_3.

Table 10-10 Common Mixed Acid-Base Disturbances

	pH	*pCO₂*	*HCO₃*	*Examples*
Metabolic acidosis Respiratory alkalosis	V	↓↓	↓	Salicylates Sepsis
Metabolic acidosis Respiratory acidosis	↓↓	↑	↓	Cardiogenic shock COPD with uremia
Metabolic acidosis Metabolic alkalosis	N	N	N	Vomiting with uremia Vomiting with diarrhea
Metabolic alkalosis Respiratory acidosis	V	↑	↑	Diuretics with COPD
Metabolic alkalosis Metabolic acidosis Respiratory alkalosis	V	V	V	Vomiting, sepsis and shock

V = variable; N = "near" normal; COPD = chronic obstructive pulmonary disease.

The presence of any of these clues should raise the possibility of a mixed disturbance.

Case 10-1: *Discussion*

1. This patient presents with a severe hyperchloremic metabolic acidosis with a normal AG. In the differential diagnosis, the hyperchloremic acidoses can be conveniently classified as a condition associated with hyperkalemia (caused by hypoaldosteronism, ACE inhibitors, potassium-sparing diuretics, and a variety of interstitial renal parenchymal diseases) or hypokalemia (caused by diarrhea, proximal or distal RTA, acetazolamide). Diarrhea is characterized by renal sodium and bicarbonate conservation (urinary sodium < 20 mEq/L; urinary pH < 6). On the other hand, RTA is associated with renal sodium and bicarbonate wastage (urinary Na > 30 mEq/L; urinary pH > 6).

2. In this patient, the diagnosis of RTA is based on the presence of an hyperchloremic (non-AG) metabolic acidosis with hypokalemia and inappropriately alkaline urine. Furthermore, because patients with proximal RTA can acidify urine (pH < 6) when severely acidotic (serum HCO_3 < 10 mEq/L), this patient likely has distal RTA.

The differential diagnosis of proximal and distal RTA is listed in Table 10-4. Sjögren's syndrome is often associated with distal RTA and is the likely cause of the condition in this patient.

3. This patient needs emergent treatment with bicarbonate, potassium, phosphorus, and subsequently, calcium. To raise the patient's serum HCO_3 to 10 mEq/L, approximately 250 mEq (7 mEq/L × 36 L TBW = 252 mEq) of bicarbonate should be administered. One should not plan to increase the serum HCO_3 to greater than 10 mEq/L acutely for fear of precipitating more severe hypokalemia or the complications of hypocalcemia (e.g., tetany, seizures) resulting from a shift from ionized to non-ionized calcium. Potassium should also be administered promptly (as KCl and KPO_4) to avoid further neuromuscular weakness and potential respiratory compromise. If the pCO_2 increases to only 15 mm Hg, the H^+ concentration will increase to 120 ($H^+ = 24\,[15 \div 3]$) and the pH will decrease to approximately 6.8.

Case 10-2: *Discussion*

1. On admission, this patient has a primary respiratory acidosis (caused by chronic obstructive pulmonary disease) and a compensatory, physiologic metabolic alkalosis. His serum is therefore slightly acidemic (pH of 7.38).

2. By the 5th postoperative day, however, he has developed a significant metabolic alkalosis (serum HCO_3 of 48 mEq/L). Since no alkali was administered to the patient, his metabolic alkalosis was generated through loss of acid, likely via gastric suction. Simultaneously, he has developed volume depletion (as determined by the physical examination) and prerenal azotemia.

The compensatory respiratory response to metabolic alkalosis is to hypoventilate and retain CO_2. The appropriate pCO_2 for a serum HCO_3 of 48 mEq/L is 50 mm Hg. Therefore the pCO_2 of 40 mm Hg in this patient represents a failure to compensate (or primary respiratory alkalosis). In this case, the respiratory alkalosis is iatrogenic because of mechanical overventilation.

3. The acidic urine (pH of 5) is inappropriate for his severe alkalemia. However, with severe volume contraction, distal tubular exchange of sodium for potassium and hydrogen will continue. Thus, despite alkalosis and hypokalemia, the kidney will excrete H^+ (pH of 5) and potassium (42 mEq/L) in order to conserve sodium (ECV). In the presence of hypokalemia and mineralocorticoid, the loss of H^+ will be even greater.

4. The initial treatment should be to adjust the mechanical ventilator to allow his pCO_2 to increase. An increase in pCO_2 to 55 mm Hg would lower the serum pH to approximately 7.55.

Next, therapy should be directed at those factors responsible for the generation (gastric suction) and maintenance (volume contraction, hypokalemia corticosteroids) of his metabolic alkalosis. H_2 receptor blockers (cimetidine, ranitidine, famotidine) will decrease both the volume and H^+ content of gastric secretions. Isotonic saline with KCl should be administered in large volumes to correct not only the metabolic alkalosis (by lowering the threshold for

HCO$_3$ reabsorption) but also the prerenal azotemia. If steroids are needed, those with minimal mineralocorticoid activity should be used.

Case 10-3: *Discussion*

1. This patient has two primary acid-base disturbances. The first is a high AG metabolic acidosis. If one assumes the normal AG to be 12, her AG of 20 requires that we account for eight additional anions. Since lactate can account for only three of these, we must search for an additional etiology as well. Beta hydroxybutyrate, methanol, ethylene glycol, and salicylates should be considered as causes. Her azotemia is probably not severe enough to totally account for the remainder of this AG.

The second primary acid-base disturbance is respiratory alkalosis. A physiologic respiratory compensation to her metabolic acidosis should only decrease the pCO$_2$ to 23 mm Hg (1.5 × 10 + 8 = 23). The patient's pCO$_2$ of 17 mm Hg indicates that primary respiratory alkalosis has also occurred. One must therefore search for a possible etiology for respiratory alkalosis such as hypoxemia, hepatic failure, sepsis, salicylates, or a CNS disease.

2. The combination of a simultaneously occurring primary metabolic acidosis and primary respiratory alkalosis should always raise the possibility of salicylate toxicity. Indeed, this patient's salicylate level on admission was 52 mg/ml (therapeutic 10 to 20 mg/ml).

References

Adroque HJ, Barrero J, Ryan JE, Dolson GM. Diabetic keto-acidosis: a practical approach. Hosp Pract 1989; 24:83.

Cohen JJ, Kassirer JP (eds). Acid-base. Boston: Little, Brown, 1983.

Emmett M, Narins RG. Clinical use of the anion gap. Medicine 1977; 56:33.

Kassirer JP. Serious acid-base disorders. N Engl J Med 1974; 291:773.

Madias NE, Perrone PD. Acid-base disorders in association with renal disease. In: Schrier RW, Gottschalk CW, (eds). Diseases of the kidney. 4th ed. Boston: Little, Brown, 1988.

McSherry E. Renal tubular acidosis in childhood. Kidney Int 1981; 20:799.

Narins RG, Emmett M. Simple and mixed acid-base disorders: a practical approach. *Medicine* 1980; 59:161.

Rose BD. Clinical physiology of acid-base and electrolyte disorders. 3rd ed. New York: McGraw Hill, 1989.

11   Urinary Tract Infection Syndromes

- Case Presentations
- Diagnosis of Urinary Tract Infection
- Urinary Tract Infection Syndromes
- Complicated Urinary Tract Infection
- Uncomplicated Urinary Tract Infection
- Case Discussions

Case 11-1

A 28-year-old woman presented with progressive urinary frequency, urgency, and dysuria which she had had for 1 week. She had had one to two "bladder infections" every year since becoming sexually active. At the time of presentation, she had multiple sexual partners. She was otherwise healthy with no previous hospitalizations or severe illnesses.

Urinalysis showed eight to ten WBC/hpf without hematuria or bacteriuria.

Questions

1. What further history would be helpful?
2. What further tests should be ordered?
3. What is the appropriate treatment for this patient?

Case 11-2

A 70-year-old woman had recurrent flank pain, low-grade fever, and dysuria for 6 to 8 months before her admission to the hospital. Urine cultures repeatedly showed *Streptococcus faecalis*. Despite a 4-week course of treatment with appropriate antibiotics, neither her symptoms nor culture cleared. Her BUN was 42 mg/dl, and her serum creatinine level was 3.3 mg/dl. Intravenous pyelography showed bilateral renal shrinkage (left > right) with a few dilated calyces and cortical thinning.

Questions

1. What is the diagnostic implication of her relapsing urinary tract infection?
2. What further tests should be performed?

Case 11-3

A 68-year-old woman with chronic renal insufficiency caused by hypertension presented with a 24-hour history of chills and fever. Blood pressure was 90/50. WBC count was 23.5 with a left shift. Her BUN was 93 mg/dl, and her serum creatinine level was 5.3 mg/dl. Blood and urine cultures showed *Escherichia coli*. A CT scan without a contrast agent failed to show urinary obstruction or any other anatomic abnormality. Treatment with gentamicin was started with a loading dose of 2 mg/kg and a maintenance dose of 1 mg/kg every 36 hours. Peak and trough gentamicin levels were appropriate. Over the next 3 days, she improved. Fever and leukocytosis both resolved. BUN and serum creatinine improved to 62 mg/dl and 4.7 mg/dl, respectively. The gentamicin was discontinued after 12 days.

Within 1 week after treatment with the antibiotics was discontinued, fever and chills recurred. Urine culture was again positive for *E. coli*.

Questions

1. Why did the urinary tract infection recur?
2. What is the appropriate therapy for this patient?

Case 11-4

A 24-year-old woman presented with a 1-day history of frequency and dysuria. Her past medical history was completely unremarkable. According to the patient, she had had two previous "bladder infections." She denied having had fever, sweats, flank pain, nausea, vomiting, or vaginal discharge. She had her last menstrual period 1 week before the time of admission.

The physical examination was normal. Urinalysis showed ten to 14 WBC/hpf, six to ten RBC/hpf, and bacteria on sediment examination.

Questions

1. What is the most likely diagnosis?
2. What are the most likely offending organisms?
3. What further tests are needed?
4. What is the appropriate treatment for this patient?

Despite the variety of syndromes produced by infection in the genitourinary tract (pyelonephritis, cystitis, prostatitis, and ureteritis), afflicted patients usually present with similar nonspecific complaints such as urinary frequency, urgency, and dysuria. Because the therapy of such syndromes may differ considerably, symptoms alone are an insufficient basis for accurate diagnosis and treatment. However, with the clinical history and a few diagnostic tests (Table 11-1), one can apply a rational approach to the patient with a urinary tract infection.

Diagnosis of Urinary Tract Infection

For years, the urine culture has been the "gold standard" for diagnosing urinary tract infections (UTIs). In most patients with acute pyelonephritis, a midstream urine culture demonstrates more than 100,000 colonies/ml and is diagnostic of UTI in asymptomatic patients. In clinical practice, however, most UTIs are neither acute

Table 11-1 Diagnostic and Therapeutic Features of the Common UTI Syndromes

	Acute Pyelonephritis	Subclinical Pyelonephritis	Bacterial Cystourethritis	Chlamydia Urethritis	Vaginitis
History and physical	Nausea, vomiting, fever, chills, flank pain, tenderness	Recurrent (3/yr) or recent (<6 wks) UTI Diabetic or immunocompromised	Dysuria, frequency, urgency, absence of pyelonephritis symptoms or signs	Prolonged onset Sexual partner is new or has urethritis	Vaginal discharge or irritation
Typical UA	Pyuria, WBC casts, bacteriuria, hematuria, proteinuria	Pyuria, bacteriuria, hematuria	Pyuria, bacteriuria, hematuria	Pyuria, no bacteriuria or hematuria	No midstream pyuria
Bacterial culture	$>10^5$ GNR, GPC	$>10^5$ GNR, GPC	$>10^2$ GNR, GPC	Neg	Neg
Treatment	2-week course of TMP/SMZ or amoxicillin	Similar to that of patients with acute pyelonephritis	Single-dose therapy of TMP/SMZ or amoxicillin	10-day course of doxycycline or erythromycin	Specific for yeast, trichomonas, etc.

GNR = gram negative rods; GPC = gram positive cocci

pyelonephritis nor asymptomatic, and most patients have lower urinary tract symptoms (cystourethritis). Stamm and colleagues clearly demonstrated that, in these patients (i.e., symptomatic), a midstream urine culture with more than 10^2 colonies/ml is diagnostic of UTI. In fact, only 50% of symptomatic patients with documented UTI by suprapubic aspiration have colony counts of more than 10^5, whereas 95% have counts of more than 10^2.

Despite the diagnostic value of the urine culture, the clinician need not obtain one for the routine, uncomplicated UTI. Cultures add significantly to the cost of a work-up. In addition, most bacteria that are cultured (*E. coli, Proteus, Staphylococcus saprophyticus*) are sensitive to the commonly prescribed urinary antibiotics (trimethoprim-sulfamethoxazole and amoxicillin). Even those bacteria not sensitive by in vitro methods are usually sensitive in vivo because of the high concentration of these antibiotics in the urine. Therefore, although the urine culture is valuable and often necessary when one is evaluating complicated UTIs, it is no longer routinely recommended.

Rather than the urine culture, the urinalysis (UA) assumes the dominant role for the laboratory evaluation of UTIs. When properly prepared (i.e., with 10 ml of a clean catch, midstream urine centrifuged at 2,000 revolutions/min for 5 minutes with resuspension of the sediment in 0.5 ml supernatant), a urine demonstrating five or more leukocytes per hpf is highly correlated with a UTI. The UA also allows detection of bacteria, blood, and protein that can help in differentiating the various syndromes. Pyuria, for example, is seen with pyelonephritis, bacterial cystourethritis, and urethritis without vaginitis. Bacteriuria and hematuria are usually absent with chlamydial infections.

In addition to the urinary sediment examination, chemical tests to detect leukocyte esterase (released by WBCs) and nitrite (produced from dietary nitrate by bacteria) are available by dipstick method. Both are highly specific for UTI but lack sensitivity. In addition, when these tests are relied upon for diagnosis, one loses the ability to evaluate the presence of gross bacteriuria, hematuria, proteinuria, or casts. Thus, examination of the urine sediment appears to be the most practical test for the diagnosis of UTI.

The Urinary Tract Infection Syndromes

Acute Pyelonephritis

A variety of syndromes are lumped under the heading UTI. Acute pyelonephritis is characterized by a history of spiking fevers, chills, nausea, and vomiting, with unilateral or bilateral flank pain and tenderness. The UA shows pyuria, usually WBC casts, bacteriuria on unspun urine, mild proteinuria, and microhematuria. A urine culture usually shows more than 10^5 colonies/ml. An IVP or renal ultrasonogram should be obtained to exclude any complicating anatomic factor such as obstruction or stones. If there are no complications, a 2-week course of trimethoprim-sulfamethoxazole (TMP/SMZ) (320/1,600 mg/day) gives excellent results. An alternative treatment is amoxicillin, 2 g/day. A follow-up culture should be obtained to document cure 3 to 5 days after therapy has ended.

Subclinical Pyelonephritis

Some patients may have subclinical pyelonephritis. This may be found in 30 to 80% of patients presenting only with frequency, dysuria, and pyuria thought to be typical of a lower UTI. These patients are often diabetic, immunocompromised, or have a history of relapsing infection or childhood UTI. Often they have had acute pyelonephritis within the previous year. Although the optimum therapy for these patients is unknown, it should probably be the same that for patients with acute pyelonephritis. Follow-up cultures should also be obtained 3 to 5 days after treatment.

Cystourethritis

Cystourethritis, the typical bacterial lower UTI, usually involves both bladder and urethra. The most commonly involved organisms are *E. coli, Proteus mirabilis,* and *S. saprophyticus,* which usually respond to TMP/SMZ or ampicillin. Therefore cultures are usually unnecessary. These patients are usually identified by default—that is, they lack the historical, physical, or urinalysis features of the other syndromes but nevertheless have frequency, dysuria, pyuria, and bacteriuria. If the history fails to elicit previous pyelonephritis, a recent UTI relapse, structural abnormalities of the urinary tract, diabetes, or immune compromise, then a variety of single-dose or "mini-dose" antibiotic regimens are appropriate. We recommend TMP/SMZ (320 mg/1,600 mg) or amoxicillin (2 g). Although slightly less effective than traditional 7- to 10-day therapy in most series, single-dose treatment offers the advantages of lower cost, improved patient compliance, and fewer side effects. In addition, such an approach may have some diagnostic value because "failures" are more likely to have complicated or upper UTIs requiring a more aggressive diagnostic or therapeutic approach.

Chlamydia Urethritis

Chlamydia urethritis usually does not involve the bladder. Patients with this condition are often identified by a stuttering or prolonged onset of symptoms over a 7- to 10-day period. A recent change in sexual partners or a partner with urethritis is also an excellent diagnostic clue. The UA may show pyuria but, unlike patients with bacterial cystourethritis, patients with chlamydia urethritis do not have hematuria and bacteriuria. A routine bacterial culture is of little value. One treatment is doxycycline, 100 mg twice daily for 10 days. An alternative is erythromycin, 500 mg four times daily for 10 days. Single-dose therapy is not effective for chlamydia.

Urethritis can also be caused by gonococcal infections, herpes simplex, *Trichomonas,* and *Candida albicans,* all of which (with the exception of *C. albicans*) typically produce pyuria. The clinician should therefore consider these possibilities when evaluating patients with frequency and dysuria with or without a urethral discharge.

Prostatitis

Prostatitis is the most common cause of UTI in men. Acute prostatitis often produces perineal and low back pain. In addition to frequency, urgency, and dysuria, chills and fever are occasionally seen. The prostate is swollen and very tender to digital examination, and massage is contraindicated. Most urologists recommend treatment with TMP/SMZ (160 mg/800 mg twice daily) for 30 days. Since UTIs in men without prostatitis rarely occur in the absence of an anatomic abnormality, males with dysuria and pyuria without symptoms or signs of prostatitis should undergo IVP with voiding and postvoid films.

Vaginitis

Although not producing pyuria in a properly collected midstream UA, vaginitis often causes frequency and dysuria. The patient should always be questioned about symptoms of discharge or vaginal irritation, and if these are present, a pelvic examination should be performed. Concomitant purulent cervicitis suggests gonococcal or chlamydial infection.

Complicated Urinary Tract Infection

Although the vast majority of UTIs are uncomplicated and rarely lead to significant long-term renal damage, the clinician must continually be alert for those unique syndromes with UTI that require aggressive diagnosis and treatment.

Complicated UTIs are those associated with immune compromise or anatomic changes within the urinary tract. These latter changes include foreign bodies (stones, stents, catheters), structural abnormalities (bladder outlet obstruction, vesicoureteral reflux, megaureter, ureteropelvic junction obstruction, or neurogenic bladder. These patients require cultures, radiographic studies, and often cystoscopy to diagnose and treat the condition adequately (see Chapter 1). *Unless clear evidence exists for prostatitis, all males with a UTI are assumed to have "complicated UTI."* Single-dose therapy is not appropriate for these patients.

Recurrent Urinary Tract Infection

Recurrent UTIs without prostatitis in men or structural abnormality in women are thought to arise by relapse of a previous inadequately treated UTI, or more commonly, by reinfection with coliform bacteria bound to vaginal and periurethral tissues. The latter can be effectively treated by continuous prophylaxis (trimethoprim, 50 to 100 mg/day) or by intermittent self-administered antibiotics (TMP/SMZ, 80 mg/400 mg/day) after sexual intercourse or for acute urinary tract symptoms. Both approaches are cost-effective for women who have three or more recurrences yearly. *It must be stressed that patients with such frequent recurrences are at high risk for having an underlying urinary tract abnormality and should undergo repeated cultures (to establish relapse or reinfection), and urologic examination.*

Catheter-Related Urinary Tract Infection

Infection commonly accompanies indwelling *bladder catheters.* In fact, virtually all catheters left in place for more than 30 days carry infection. Generally the infection is asymptomatic and remains so as long as the catheter remains unobstructed and the urinary tract is free of any other anatomic abnormality. Antibiotic therapy is not routinely recommended for patients with indwelling catheters. Antibacterials not only fail to prevent infection in this setting, but lead to infection with yeast or resistant bacteria. Symptomatic infections, particularly those leading to sepsis, should be aggressively treated with at least 2 weeks of antibiotic therapy and change of the urinary catheter. In patients with repeated septic episodes, a case for long-term suppressive antibiotics (nitrofurantoin or TMP/SMZ) to inhibit bacterial growth can be made. Sterile insertion technique and a closed dependent drainage system is always indicated for indwelling bladder catheters.

Asymptomatic Bacteriuria

Asymptomatic bacteriuria is common in young women and elderly patients of both sexes. Therapy should not be used routinely. Asymptomatic bacteriuria is often intermittent and frequently resolves spontaneously. In the absence of an underlying structural or anatomic change, there is no evidence of progressive renal damage. In addition, despite the higher mortality in elderly patients with asymptomatic bacteriuria, treatment does not appear to improve survival. Finally, antibiotics increase the toxicity; selection of resistant organisms, and cost of care in these patients.

In specific cases of asymptomatic bacteriuria, antibiotics are recommended. These are (1) pregnancy, where treatment will decrease the incidence of acute pyelonephritis and fetal mortality, (2) the presence of anatomic abnormalities such as vesicoureteral reflux or neurogenic bladder, (3) planned instrumentation of the urinary tract, or (4) struvite or calcium phosphate nephrolithiasis, where alkaline pH from urease-producing bacteria may contribute to stone growth.

Urinary Tract Infection With Renal Failure

Treatment of UTI in patients with renal failure or renal insufficiency may be difficult. As renal function diminishes, the ability to achieve adequate renal parenchymal and urinary antibiotic levels declines. This is particularly true of drugs such as aminoglycosides which rely on glomerular filtration for renal clearance. Tubular secretion of drugs such as penicillins, cephalosporins, and sulfonamides) is better maintained. In addition, the dosage adjustments needed to prevent systemic drug accumulation and toxicity often lead to inadequate urinary levels. Therefore, three principles for the treatment of UTI in patients with renal failure should be kept in mind: (1) antibiotics should be used with a large therapeutic:toxic ratio, (2) the usual dose should be prescribed (i.e., nonrenal failure dose), and (3) drugs relying on tubular secretion for renal excretion should be used. These are the penicillins, cephalosporins, and sulfonamides. One should avoid administering antibiotics cleared by glomerular filtration (aminoglycosides) or those metabolized by the liver (chloramphenicol, erythromycin, nitrofurantoin) in this situation.

Uncomplicated Urinary Tract Infection

For the patient with uncomplicated UTI (absence of underlying urinary tract disease or immune suppression) and without the unique problems outlined in the preceding section, a diagnostic and therapeutic approach is outlined in Figure 11-1.

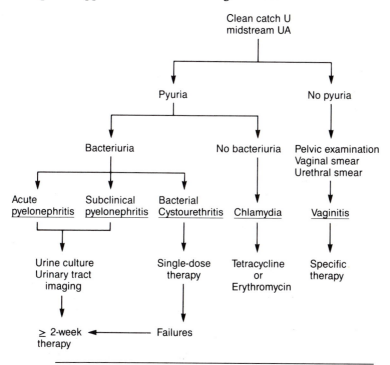

Figure 11-1: An approach to the patient with symptoms suggestive of uncomplicated UTI.

The key to the diagnostic algorithm is the presence or absence of pyuria. Vaginitis rarely produces pyuria in a properly collected midstream urine specimen, and the patient should be questioned specifically about vaginal symptoms. A pelvic examination and wet mount should then be performed and specific therapy initiated, depending on the microscopic findings (e.g., yeast, *Trichomonas*).

If pyuria is present but hematuria and bacteriuria are absent, chlamydia urethritis is a likely diagnosis, particularly if the patient's history reveals the stuttering onset of symptoms over a 7- to 10-day period or a recent change in sexual partners. Other forms of urethritis (gonococcal, herpetic) should be considered in these patients, as well. A 10-day course of a tetracycline such as doxycycline is appropriate for patients with chlamydia urethritis.

The presence of bacteriuria on unspun urine and/or WBC casts suggests acute pyelonephritis. If the clinical history (see Table 11-1) suggests acute or subclinical pyelonephritis, an IVP (or an ultrasonogram) and urine culture should be obtained. If the clinical picture does not suggest pyelonephritis but bacteria and pyuria are present, the symptomatic patient usually has bacterial cystourethritis. A urine culture is usually unnecessary. Single-dose therapy is usually effective. Patients who fail to respond to single-dose therapy should be treated as though they have pyelonephritis.

Case 11-1: *Discussion*

1. Dysuria, frequency, and urgency may result from several UTI syndromes (see Table 11-1). The gradual onset of symptoms and the absence of hematuria are suggestive of chlamydia urethritis. A history of a recent change in sexual partners or a partner with urethritis are also typical of this syndrome. Symptoms of pyelonephritis should be absent, as should bacteriuria on UA.

2. In a woman with a clinical presentation suggesting chlamydia urethritis, further diagnostic tests are unnecessary. However, the clinician must take care to exclude other causes of urethritis such as yeast and herpetic or gonococcal urethritis. A bacterial urine culture would be negative and is not necessary.

3. A treatment for chlamydia urethritis is doxycycline, 100 mg twice daily for 10 days. Her sexual partner should also be examined and treated.

Case 11-2: *Discussion*

1. An invasive UTI (pyelonephritis) is suggested by this patient's fever and flank pain. The fact that it has repeatedly relapsed despite adequate treatment suggests an underlying anatomic abnormality of the urinary tract.

2. Cystoscopy should be performed. In this patient, the results of this test were normal. Although IVP failed to demonstrate an anatomic problem, her relapsing course made this such a strong possibility that a CT scan was performed. The CT scan showed bilateral renal stones, which were missed (even in retrospect) on the IVP. The stones are probably responsible for the relapsing UTI.

A radiographic study is important to evaluate patients with pyelonephritis or recurrent UTI. Usually an IVP with voiding and postvoid films will suffice. Nevertheless, if a patient fails to clear the infection despite adequate therapy, cystoscopy and CT scanning or ultrasonography are indicated.

Case 11-3: *Discussion*

1. This case demonstrates the difficulty of treating UTI in patients with underlying renal insufficiency or renal failure. When the serum creatinine is significantly elevated (low GFR), drugs excreted by glomerular filtration, such as aminoglycosides, may not achieve adequate therapeutic levels in the urine or renal parenchyma. In this patient, the systemic sepsis resolved with aminoglycoside treatment, but the UTI recurred—probably because of inadequate urinary antibiotic levels.

2. Drugs secreted by the renal tubules are generally more effective in this setting. Thus, treatment with penicillin or a cephalosporin would be most appropriate. In order to insure adequate tissue and urinary levels, the usual dosage adjustment for renal failure should be abandoned and these drugs prescribed in their usual dosages.

Case 11-4: *Discussion*

1. In this patient with dysuria, the presence of pyuria and absence of vaginal symptoms sufficiently exclude vaginitis. The presence of hematuria and bacteriuria on the urine sediment examination makes chlamydia urethritis unlikely, as well. Neither do the history or physical examination support pyelonephritis, acute or subclinical. The most likely diagnosis is therefore a bacterial lower UTI cystourethritis.

2. *E. coli, Proteus* and *S. saprophyticus* are the most common pathogens causing cystourethritis.

3. No further diagnostic tests are needed in this patient. If, however, one chose to obtain a urine culture, a colony count of greater than 10^2 should be considered significant in this symptomatic patient.

4. Single-dose therapy for this uncomplicated UTI offers several advantages. These include improved patient compliance, cost savings, and fewer side effects. TMP/SMZ (320 mg/1,600 mg) or ampicillin (2 g) are the most popular treatments. Should the patient fail single-dose therapy, a 2-week antibiotic course is appropriate.

References

Fihn SD, Johnson L, Roberts PL, et al. Trimethoprim-sulfamethoxasole for acute dysuria in women: a single-dose or 10-day course. Ann Intern Med 1988; 108:350–357.

Komaroff AL. Acute dysuria in women. N Engl J Med 1984; 310:368–374.

Komaroff AL. Urinalysis and urine culture in women with dysuria. Ann Intern Med 1986; 104:212–218.

Nordenstam GR, Brandberg CA, Odén CS, et al. Bacteriuria and mortality in an elderly population. N Engl J Med 1986; 314:1152–1156.

Stamm WE, Counts GW, Running K, et al. Diagnosis of coliform infection in acutely dysuric women. N Engl J Med 1982; 307:463–468.

Stamm WE, McKevitt M, Counts GW. Acute renal infection in women: treatment with trimethoprim-sulfamethoxasole or ampicillin for two or six weeks. Ann Intern Med 1987; 106:341–345.

Wong ES, McKevitt M, Running K, et al. Management of recurrent urinary tract infections with patient-administered single-dose therapy. Ann Intern Med 1985; 102:302–307.

12 Nephrolithiasis

- Case Presentations

- Principles of Stone Formation

- Causes of Nephrolithiasis

- Evaluation of the Patient

- Diagnostic Approach

- Case Discussions

Case 12-1

A 36-year-old female presented to the emergency room with left flank pain and hematuria. An IVP was obtained (Fig. 12-1). She was admitted for pain control and forced hydration and shortly thereafter passed a stone. Analysis of the stone showed calcium oxalate.

Family history revealed that her father and brother had had recurrent nephrolithiasis. Past medical history revealed that the patient had had a similar episode of pain on the right side at age 16 years which was diagnosed as "appendicitis." No surgery was performed. She weighed 55 kg at the time of the episode.

Serum calcium, phosphorus, urea, creatinine, and electrolytes were normal. The urine sample collected over a 24-hour period

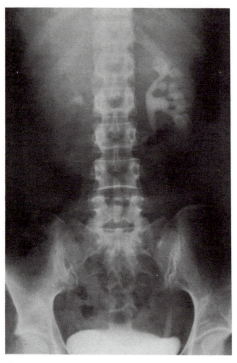

Figure 12-1: *A,* Intravenous pyelogram in patient of Case 12-1.

A

revealed 112 mg of calcium, 20 mg of oxalate, 301 mg of uric acid, 553 mg of citrate, and a creatinine clearance rate of 121 ml/min. Urine volume was 600 ml/24 hr. The urinalysis was completely normal with a pH of 5.5, and revealed no cells.

Questions

1. What is the cause of calcium lithiasis in this patient?
2. What is the appropriate treatment?

Case 12-2

A 24-year-old male reported having passed several kidney stones over the past 36 months. He was told that the most recent stone was calcium oxalate. Several small radiopaque stones re-

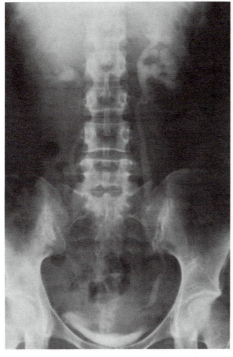

Figure 12-1: B, Intravenous pyelogram in patient of Case 12-1.
Figure continues on following page.

B

mained in the renal pelvis, as demonstrated by a plain film of his abdomen.

Past treatment with a low-calcium diet, high-fluid intake, and thiazide diuretics had failed to control his nephrolithiasis.

Outpatient evaluation showed normal blood chemistries. A urine sample collected over a 24-hour period showed 166 mg of calcium, 24 mg of oxalate, 1,150 mg of uric acid, 463 mg of citrate and a creatinine clearance rate of 98 ml/min. UA showed a pH of 6.5, SG of 1.022, and a normal sediment.

Questions

1. What is the cause of his recurrent calcium lithiasis?
2. How should it be treated?

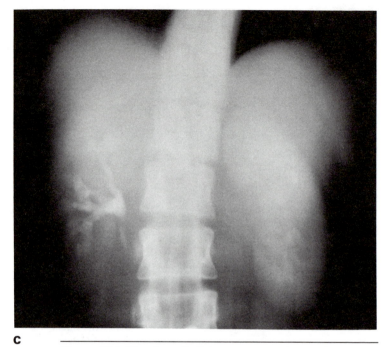

C

Figure 12-1 (Continued): C, Intravenous pyelogram in patient of Case 12-1.

Case 12-3

A 46-year-old female was admitted with right flank pain 2 days after undergoing extracorporeal shock wave lithotripsy (ESWL) for right nephrolithiasis. X-ray examination revealed right ureteral obstruction caused by numerous opaque stone fragments. The obstruction was relieved by percutaneous nephrostomy and endoscopic removal of stone fragments.

She had had recurrent nephrolithiasis that required seven major operations during the previous 8 years. She had also undergone "bowel surgery" for Crohn's disease 20 years earlier. Review of systems revealed that she passed six to ten loose stools per day.

Serum chemistries revealed Na of 142 mEq/L, K of 3.2 mEq/L, Cl of 112 mEq/L, HCO_3 of 21 mEq/L, and normal calcium, phosphorus, and uric acid. UA showed a pH of 5, SG of 1.016 with microhematuria, and four to six WBC/hpf. Urine culture was negative; a urine sample collected over a 24-hour period showed 104 mg of calcium, 232 mg of oxalate, 206 mg of uric acid, 484 mg of citrate, and a creatinine clearance rate of 54 ml/min.

Questions

1. What is the cause of recurrent nephrolithiasis in this patient?
2. What is the appropriate therapy?

An underlying metabolic or anatomic defect can be identified in most patients with nephrolithiasis. In addition, there is specific therapy for many causes of renal stone formation. Thus, a comprehensive evaluation is necessary in any patient with nephrolithiasis.

Principles of Stone Formation

Stone formation occurs when the urinary concentration of a substance exceeds its solubility. This may be due to supersaturation of the urine, a deficiency of various inhibitors to stone formation, or the presence of factors potentiating stone formation (Table 12-1).

Urinary supersaturation caused by excessive excretion of various substances (calcium, oxalate, uric acid, or cystine) may be solely responsible for stone formation in some cases. A low urine volume may contribute to supersaturation by raising the urinary concentration of a given substance. In other situations, a change in urinary pH may affect the solubility. For example, at similar urinary concentrations, uric acid and cystine stones are more likely to form in acid urine, whereas calcium phosphate and struvite stones are more likely to form in alkaline urine.

Citrate, by binding calcium and forming a very soluble salt, serves as a major inhibitor to renal stone formation and growth. There are numerous other inhibitors to stone formation. A defi-

Table 12-1 Causes of Nephrolithiasis

Supersaturation of urine
  Excess excretion
    Hypercalciuria
    Hyperoxaluria
    Hyperuricosuria
    Hypercystinuria
  Decreased urine volume
  Change in urine pH
    Acid (uric acid and cystine stone)
    Alkali (calcium phosphate and struvite stones)

Deficiency of inhibitors to stone formation
  Hypocitraturia
  Low urinary pyrophosphate
  Others

Potentiation of stone formation
  Infection (Urea-splitting bacteria)
  Stasis (MSK, infundibular stenosis, ureteropelvic junction obstruction, primary obstructive megaureter)

ciency of one or more of these inhibitors will promote crystallization and/or augment stone growth at any given urine concentration.

In some patients, infection or anatomic changes may potentiate stone formation. At a given concentration of urinary calcium, calcium phosphate stones are more likely to form in a patient infected with urea-splitting organisms. Similarly, by causing slow flow in ectatic terminal collecting tubules, medullary sponge kidney potentiates calcium lithiasis. Uric acid crystalluria may promote the formation of calcium stones by serving as a nidus for calcium precipitation.

Thus, in any patient with nephrolithiasis, one must consider the possibility of urinary supersaturation, a decrement in the inhibitor citrate, urinary infection, and MSK.

Causes of Nephrolithiasis

Table 12-2 outlines the various types of renal stones, their pathophysiology, major causes and primary treatments. Calcium stones account for roughly 75% of cases, followed by struvite

(15%), uric acid (8%), cystine (1 to 2%), and miscellaneous causes such as triamterene and xanthine stones (1 to 2%).

Calcium Oxalate Stones

Most calcium stones are calcium oxalate. They are radiopaque on a plain film of the abdomen. They may occur in patients with urinary supersaturation of calcium, oxalate, or uric acid (where a uric acid crystal serves as a nidus for stone growth) or in patients with hypocitraturia (deficient inhibitor).

Hypercalciuria

Hypercalciuria (>4 mg/kg/24 hr) can occur with or without hypercalcemia (Tables 12-3 and 12-4, respectively). If hypercalcemia exists, treatment should focus on the underlying disease. With idiopathic hypercalciuria (whether absorptive or renal leak), thiazide-type diuretics (hydrochlorothiazide 12.5 to 25 mg every 12 hours, or chlorthalidone, 25 mg daily) are indicated as primary therapy. These agents cause mild extracellular volume contraction, thus stimulating renal tubular calcium reabsorption and lowering urinary calcium. By binding intestinal calcium and raising the level of urinary inhibitors (citrate and pyrophosphate), orthophosphates (Neutra-Phos 60 to 90 ml, three times daily, or Neutra-Phos-K, two tablets three times daily) are also effective in treating calcium lithiasis caused by idiopathic hypercalciuria.

Hyperoxaluria

Hyperoxaluria may be a primary genetic defect (hereditary hyperoxaluria), albeit rarely. Although the results are usually unsatisfactory, these patients can be treated with orthophosphates or magnesium oxide, which competitively bind both urinary oxalate, thus increasing solubility, and intestinal oxalate, thus limiting absorption. More commonly, hyperoxaluria is caused by intestinal oxalate hyperabsorption associated with the fat malabsorption of regional enteritis, intestinal bypass surgery, and other short bowel syndromes. Here, intestinal calcium preferentially binds to fat,

Table 12-2 Mechanisms, Causes, and Treatments of the Common Renal Stones

Stone	Mechanism	Cause	Therapy
Calcium*			
Calcium oxalate	Hypercalciuria	Hypercalcemia	Treat underlying cause
		Hypercalciuria	Thiazides
			Orthophosphates
	Hyperoxaluria	Primary (genetic)	Orthophosphates
			Magnesium oxide
		Enteric	Low-fat/oxalate diet, oral calcium
			Cholestyramine
	Hyperuricosuria	Idiopathic	Allopurinol
	Hypocitraturia	Idiopathic	Oral citrate
			Orthophosphates
		Secondary (RTA, UTI, acidosis)	Treat underlying condition
Calcium phosphate	Hypercalciuria	Hypercalciuria	Thiazides
	Urinary stasis	Medullary sponge kidney	Thiazides
			Orthophosphates
	Alkaline urine	RTA	Treat infection
			Surgery

Type	Urine	Cause	Treatment
Struvite[†]			
Magnesium ammonium phosphate	Alkaline urine	Infection	Treat infection Surgery Acetohydroxamic acid (Lithostat)
Uric acid[‡]	Hyperuricosuria	Hyperuricemia Idiopathic	Allopurinol Allopurinol Low-purine (protein) diet Alkali to urinary pH 6–7
Cystine[§]	Acid urine Cystinuria	Low urinary ammonia Genetic defect	Urinary volume 4 L/day Alkali to urinary pH >7.5 Penicillamine
Miscellaneous[§]			
Triamterene	6-p-Hydroxytriamterene	Triamterene	Discontinue drug
Xanthine	Xanthinuria	Hereditary	Urine volume 4 L/day Alkali
Oxypurinol		Allopurinol High-dose allopurinol	Discontinue drug Discontinue drug

*Accounts for 75% of cases.
†Accounts for 15% of cases.
‡Accounts for 8% of cases.
§Accounts for 1–2% of cases.

Table 12-3 Hypercalciuria With Hypercalcemia

Hyperparathyroidism	Milk alkali syndrome
Malignancy	Paget's disease
Sarcoidosis	Immobilization
Vitamin D intoxication	

leaving oxalate free for absorption in the colon. Treatment is thus aimed at decreasing "free" intestinal oxalate by dietary oxalate restriction (Table 12-5) and enteric binding of oxalate (with a high-calcium, low-fat diet and supplemental oral calcium, 500 mg twice daily). Cholestyramine may also be used to bind enteric fat, decreasing free oxalate and colonic absorption.

Hyperuricosuria

Patients with hyperuricosuria (>800 mg/day in males; >700 mg/day in females) may develop calcium lithiasis if uric acid crystals serve as a nidus for calcium deposition. These patients often have normal urinary calcium and oxalate excretion. Treatment is with allopurinol, 200 to 300 mg daily.

Hypocitraturia

Finally, calcium oxalate lithiasis is frequently associated with low urinary citrate excretion. Hypocitraturia (<400 mg/day in

Table 12-4 Hypercalciuria Without Hypercalcemia

Idiopathic (absorptive, renal calcium leak, renal phosphorus leak)	Malignancy
RTA (distal)	Furosemide
Sarcoidosis	Paget's disease
Medullary sponge kidney	Immobilization

Table 12-5 Major Dietary Sources of Oxalate

Rhubarb	Chocolate
Spinach	Cocoa
Beet greens	Tea
Turnip greens	Grapefruit juice
Sweet potatoes	Orange juice
Nuts	Cranberry juice

males; <500 mg/day in females) is usually idiopathic and particularly common in females. Oral citrate (Urocit-K, three tablets three times daily, or Polycitra-K, 15 ml three times daily) increases urinary citrate, which binds urinary calcium, thus inhibiting crystal growth. Orthophosphates also increase urinary citrate and may be adjunctive therapy. In some cases, hypocitraturia may be secondary to an underlying condition such as renal tubular acidosis, urinary infection, chronic diarrhea with metabolic acidosis, and hypokalemia. In this situation, treatment is centered on the primary disease.

In most patients with calcium lithiasis, the ratio of urinary citrate (mg/l) to calcium (mg/l) best identifies the propensity to stone formation. Urine citrate: calcium is usually less than 4 in female stone-formers, and less than 3 in males.

Calcium Phosphate Stones

Calcium phosphate stones may form in patients with hypercalciuria alone but are usually seen with alkaline urine due to infection with urea-splitting bacteria. In the former, thiazides will suffice; in the latter, eradicating the underlying infection is most important. Often, urologic intervention (e.g., surgery, ESWL, percutaneous nephrolithotomy, ureteroscopy) will be necessary to accomplish this goal. Distal RTA may cause hypocitraturia, hypercalciuria, and an alkaline urine and should be excluded in all patients with calcium lithiasis—particularly calcium phosphate lithiasis. Finally, calcium phosphate lithiasis may complicate roughly 15% of patients with medullary sponge kidney. Cystic dilation of the terminal collecting tubules results in slow urine flow. Hypercalciuria may be present in some. Both thiazides and orthophosphates are effective in stone-formers with MSK.

Struvite Stones

Struvite stones, which account for approximately 15% of renal stones, are composed of magnesium ammonium phosphate (triple phosphate). They are radiopaque and usually form a large homogeneous mass in the renal pelvis and calyces (staghorn calculus). Struvite stones precipitate and grow in the presence of chronic urinary infection with urease-producing bacteria (*Proteus, Klebsiella, Pseudomonas, Staphylococcus,* and *Serratia,* but not *E. coli*). Urease splits urea-forming ammonium and hydroxyl ions, raising the urinary pH and potentiating struvite growth. Since stone growth often incorporates bacteria, surgical removal is usually necessary to eradicate the infection. Although acetohydroxamic acid (Lithostat), a urease inhibitor, may arrest and over a period of months to years dissolve struvite stones, gastrointestinal side effects limit its efficacy.

Uric Acid Stones

Uric acid stones are radiolucent. They account for 5 to 10% of renal stone disease. Hyperuricosuria is the most common cause and is usually caused by hyperuricemia in patients with gout, Lesch-Nyhan syndrome, or hypercatabolic states such as tumor lysis after chemotherapy. Hyperuricosuria without hyperuricemia can also occur. Regardless of the cause, allopurinol (100 to 300 mg daily) and a low-purine diet are recommended therapies for uric acid lithiasis when hyperuricosuria (>800 mg/day in males; >700 mg/day in females) is documented. However, nearly half of the patients with uric acid stones have a normal urinary uric acid excretion. In most of these patients, a low urine pH contributes to stone formation by decreasing uric acid solubility. Oral alkali (25 to 75 mEq daily) will usually raise urinary pH to 6 or 7 and effectively treat uric acid stones.

Cystinuria

Cystinuria is a rare autosomal recessive defect responsible for 1 to 2% of patients with nephrolithiasis. Cystine stones are usually radiopaque but may initially be radiolucent. The diagnosis can be suspected by demonstrating the characteristic hexagonal crystals in the urine (present in only 20% of the patients) or a positive qualitative cystine screen on the urine. Documenting increased cystine excretion in a urine sample collected over a 24-hour period (>400 mg daily) confirms the diagnosis. Increasing urine volume to greater than 4 L per day and alkalinizing the urine to a pH of more than 7.5 will effectively treat approximately one-third of cystine stone-formers. In the remainder, penicillamine reduces urinary cystine excretion and usually dissolves cystine stones.

Miscellaneous Causes

Other causes include xanthine stones which may result from hereditary xanthinuria or allopurinol therapy in patients with extreme hyperuricemia. High urine volume and alkali therapy is usually effective. High-dose allopurinol therapy can also result in oxypurinol stones. Triamterene is another drug occasionally responsible for nephrolithiasis. The treatment for these drug-related renal stones is simply to discontinue the drug.

Evaluation of the Patient

In any patient with nephrolithiasis, one must assess both surgical and metabolic activity. Surgically active stones are those associated with infection (particularly systemic infections), obstruction, pain, or major hematuria.

Urologic Approach to Nephrolithiasis

The open surgical approach to nephrolithiasis is not widely practiced because of the availability of ESWL, percutaneous stone removal, and manipulative treatment with fluoroscopy and endoscopy. If severe obstruction or sepsis is present, urinary drainage can be provided by percutaneous nephrostomy or retrograde passage of a ureteral catheter.

The principles of ESWL are the localization of the stone(s) by two-dimensional radiographic scanning or ultrasonography and focusing shock waves produced by electrodes onto the targeted stone(s) through a water bath or water bag. After the stones are fragmented, the small particles are passed in the urine during the next few weeks. It is common for a ureteral stent to be passed cystoscopically before ESWL to prevent renal obstruction by stone fragments. The ideal stone for treatment with ESWL is one that is not infected, is located in the renal pelvis, and is less than 3 cm in diameter. Contraindications to the procedure are active UTI and urinary tract obstruction. Patients with ureteral calculi have also been successfully treated with ESWL, and the success rate is sufficient to make ESWL the first-line treatment for most upper urinary tract calculi.

Percutaneous nephrostolithotomy involves removal of renal and proximal ureteral calculi through a nephroscope that has been inserted through a nephrostomy tract. An ultrasound probe can be used to fragment calculi that are too large to be extracted through the nephrostomy tract. Combined percutaneous and ESWL therapy for staghorn calculi is an alternative to anatrophic nephrolithotomy. Percutaneous nephrostolithotomy with ultrasonic lithotripsy is used to fragment and extract as much of the stone burden as possible. If the kidney is stone-free, the treatment goal has been accomplished. If the stone remnants are smaller than 5 mm in diameter, they may be extracted with a flexible nephroscope or allowed to pass down the stented ureter spontaneously. If after percutaneous nephrostolithotomy the stone remnants are larger than 5 mm in diameter, ESWL is applied, followed a few days later by flexible nephroscopy and percutaneous removal of residual stone fragments, if necessary.

Open surgical removal of upper urinary tract calculi is indicated when percutaneous or ESWL techniques fail or when multiple or branched calculi are associated with obstruction that must be surgically corrected.

Nearly all ureteral calculi that are smaller than 5 mm in diameter will pass spontaneously with expectant management consisting of hydration and analgesics. The indications for hospital admission and surgical or manipulative treatment are urinary tract sepsis, severe colic that is unresponsive to oral medication, severe nausea and vomiting, complete ureteral obstruction, or stone impaction.

Distal ureteral stones are best managed by ureteroscopic stone manipulation or stone-basketing. Mid- and upper ureteral calculi that are small may be removed endoscopically with stone catheters and fluoroscopy guidance. Open surgical stone removal is necessary only in patients who do not respond to expectant or manipulative therapy and ESWL.

Medical Approach

Metabolically active stone disease is defined as documented stone growth or the passage of "gravel" during the previous 12 months. Patients who are "inactive" require only the general "stone clinic advice" (Table 12-6) and periodic follow-up radiographs (KUB or IVP). Patients who are "active" require more aggressive and specific treatment, depending on the underlying metabolic derangement responsible for stone formation (see Table 12-2). In the metabolic evaluation, therefore, one must assess all

Table 12-6 "Stone Clinic Advice": General Advice for All Patients With Nephrolithiasis

Maintain urine volume at >2 L/day

Restrict dietary sodium to <120 mEq/day

Restrict dietary protein/purine

Avoid loop diuretics and triamterene

Table 12-7 Diagnostic Protocol to Evaluate Patients With Nephrolithiasis

Tests	Day 1	2	3
Serum			
Calcium	✔		✔
Phosphorus	✔		✔
Electrolytes*	✔		✔
Uric acid	✔		✔
BUN	✔		✔
Creatinine	✔		✔
Urine			
Creatinine clearance		✔	✔
Calcium (mg/24 hr)		✔	✔
Oxalate (mg/24 hr)		✔	✔
Uric acid (mg/24 hr)		✔	✔
Citrate (mg/24 hr)		✔	✔
Sodium (mEq/24 hr)		✔	✔
Cystine (qualitative)[†]		✔	
UA[‡]	✔		

*Hyperchloremic metabolic acidosis should alert one to RTA.
[†]Positive cystine screen necessitates 24-hour urine cystine.
[‡]Pyuria necessitates urine culture; a pH of > 6 requires further evaluation for infection or RTA.

potential mechanisms responsible for stone formation as outlined in Table 12-1.

Table 12-7 outlines a protocol for initial urine- and blood-testing in a patient with nephrolithiasis. Testing can be easily performed on an outpatient basis, with the patient receiving his usual diet; in fact, this is the preferred setting.

Positive screening tests can be verified by more specific testing— for example, 24-hour urinary cystine if qualitative cystine screen is positive, or urine culture if pyuria is present on UA.

Diagnostic Approach

Based on the above pathophysiologic and treatment considerations, a diagnostic and therapeutic approach to nephrolithiasis is outlined in Figure 12-2. One must first assess the surgical activity of the patient's stone disease and then treat it accordingly. For nonsurgical stone disease, one should determine the metabolic basis for stone formation. This is accomplished by the testing protocol outlined in Table 12-7. As mentioned, in most patients with nephrolithiasis, an underlying metabolic derangement is uncovered. Appropriate therapy (as outlined in Table 12-2 and Figure 12-2) depends on its identification.

Case 12-1: *Discussion*

1. This patient with severe pain was initially treated in the hospital, but shortly thereafter became a "nonsurgical" problem after passing a stone. The patient now requires a medical evaluation to determine the metabolic basis for her underlying stone disease (see Fig. 12-2).

A complete evaluation was performed as outlined in Table 12-7. This failed to show urinary supersaturation with calcium, oxalate, or uric acid. Similarly, she had no evidence of hypocitraturia, thus ruling out (in most cases) a deficient inhibitor as the cause of the stone disease. The UA appeared to exclude RTA and UTI as contributing factors.

Since no underlying mechanism for her calcium stone disease was apparent, a close review of her initial IVP was performed (Fig. 12-1). This revealed evidence of MSK, which can contribute to stone disease by causing slow urinary flow through the distal collecting tubules.

In approximately 15% of patients, MSK is hereditary. This may explain the strong family history of nephrolithiasis in this patient.

2. If the patient did not have medullary sponge kidney, one could argue for observation and no specific therapy other than "stone clinic advice." With the potential for recurrent nephrolithiasis caused by the anatomic defect of medullary sponge kidney, however, further treatment is probably indicated. Thiazide diuretics

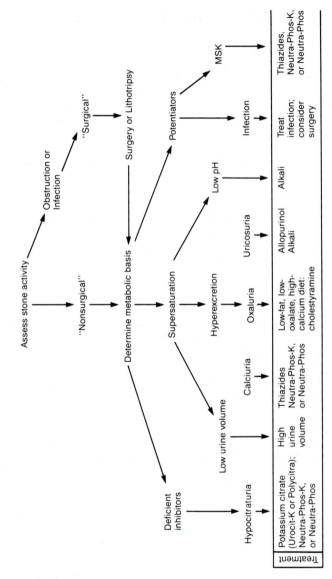

Assess stone activity

→ Obstruction or Infection → "Surgical" → Surgery or Lithotripsy

→ "Nonsurgical" → Determine metabolic basis

Determine metabolic basis branches to:

- Deficient inhibitors → Hypocitraturia → **Treatment:** Potassium citrate (Urocit-K or Polycitra); Neutra-Phos-K, or Neutra-Phos
- Low urine volume → High urine volume
- Supersaturation

Supersaturation branches to:

- Calciuria → Thiazides Neutra-Phos-K, or Neutra-Phos
- Hyperexcretion
  - Oxaluria → Low-fat, low-oxalate, high-calcium diet; cholestyramine
  - Uricosuria → Allopurinol Alkali
- Low pH → Alkali
- Potentiators
  - Infection → Treat infection; consider surgery
  - MSK → Thiazides, Neutra-Phos-K, or Neutra-Phos

Treatment

314

will decrease urinary calcium excretion and aid in therapy. In addition, oral phosphate therapy may also have a therapeutic effect by decreasing urinary calcium.

Case 12-2: *Discussion*

1. Similar to the patient in Case 12-1, this young man has nonsurgical stone disease.

The outpatient evaluation to determine the metabolic basis for his stone disease (see Table 12-7) revealed a significantly high urinary uric acid excretion (1,150 mg/24 hr). The other potential factors for supersaturation, such as hypercalciuria or hyperoxaluria, could not be documented, despite the documentation of previous calcium oxalate stones.

The underlying cause of this patient's calcium lithiasis is most likely hyperuricosuria. By forming a nidus for calcification, uric acid crystals can predispose to recurrent calcium lithiasis. This may be an occult cause of calcium lithiasis in a significant number of patients.

2. The patient should be treated with allopurinol, 100 to 300 mg/day.

Case 12-3: *Discussion*

1. Initially, this patient was admitted to the hospital for surgical stone disease. Her right ureteral obstruction was treated successfully by percutaneous drainage and her acute problems resolved.

After surgical correction of her problem, a metabolic stone workup was undertaken (see Table 12-7). This revealed a striking elevation of urinary oxalate, indicating that hyperoxaluria was likely the cause of her recurrent calcium lithiasis.

Her age and negative family history, however, exclude primary hyperoxaluria as a cause. Rather, her oxaluria is probably caused by increased intestinal oxalate absorption due to her short bowel syndrome. Because of the constant steatorrhea and calcium saponification in her bowel, enteric oxalate was left "free" for absorption from

◄ **Figure 12-2:** Diagnostic and therapeutic approach to patients with nephrolithiasis.

the gut and eventual urinary excretion. Calcium oxalate lithiasis is a common long-term complication of short bowel syndromes from any cause (e.g., previous intestinal bypass surgery, Crohn's disease).

2. The appropriate treatment is cholestyramine, one-half packet twice daily. In this patient, it markedly decreased not only her urinary oxalate excretion but also her diarrhea (for which she was very grateful). In addition, she was to receive a low-oxalate diet supplemented with oral calcium. During the subsequent 3 years, no evidence of new stone formation was discovered.

References

Ettinger B, Tang A, Citron JT, et al. Randomized trial of allopurinol in the prevention of calcium oxalate calculi. N Engl J Med 1986; 315:1386–1389.

Pak CYC. Medical management of nephrolithiasis. J Urol 1982; 128:1157–1164.

Pak CYC, Fuller L. Idiopathic hypocitraturia calcium-oxalate nephrolithiasis successfully treated with potassium citrate. Ann Intern Med 1986; 104:33–37.

Parks JH, Coe FL. A urinary calcium-citrate index for the evaluation of nephrolithiasis. Kidney Int 1986; 30:85–90.

Parks JH, Coe FL, Strauss AL. Calcium nephrolithiasis and medullary sponge kidney in women. N Engl J Med 1982; 306:1088–1091.

Schriver CB. Cystinuria. N Engl J Med 1986; 315:1155–1156.

Spirnak JP, Resnick MI. Urinary stones. In: Tanagho EA, McAninch JW. Smith's General Urology. San Mateo: Appleton and Lange Co., 1988:291.

Winifield HN, Clayman RV, Chaussy CG, et al. Monotherapy of staghorn renal calculi: a comparative study between percutaneous nephrolithotomy and extracorporeal shock wave lithotripsy. J Urol 1988; 139:895–903.

Index

Note: Page numbers followed by (t) indicate tables; those followed by (f) indicate figures.

A

Abdominal bruit, diagnosis of, 45, 47
Abdominal film (KUB), 1, 2t, 3
ACE inhibitor therapy, 99, 201–202, 204, 205t
Acetazolamide, in edematous therapy, 205
Acetohydroxamic acid, 308
Acetone, 17
  effect of, on serum creatinine, 59
Acid base disturbances, primary, 262–264, 263t
Acid excretion, physiologic control of, 272t
Acidosis. *See also* Renal tubular acidosis (RTA)
  hyperchloremic, 24, 42, 265, 268
  lactic, 268
  metabolic, 42, 197, 264–266, 265f, 268, 269, 270f
  organic, 265, 266–267
  respiratory, 263, 264, 264t
  uremic, 266
Acute renal failure. *See also* Renal failure
  acute azotemia
    diagnostic approach to, 66–67, 67f, 68t
    nonrenal causes of, 58–62, 59t, 60f, 61f
    postrenal, 59–61, 60f, 61f
    prerenal, 62, 63–66, 64t
  acute tubular necrosis, 73–76, 74t
  case discussions of, 83–87
  case presentations of, 53–58
  causes of, 68, 70–71t
    acute glomerulonephritis, 72
    glomerular hemodynamics, 68–69, 72

    interstitial nephritis, 72–73
    vascular diseases, 73
  common complications of, 81–82
  diagnostic approach to, 76–77
  and excess sodium, 200-1
  factors responsible for maintenance of, 76t
  prevention of, 77–79, 78t
  treatment and prognosis of, 80, 80t
    oliguria versus nonoliguria, 81
    specific therapy for, 83
    supportive care for, 82–83
  versus prerenal azotemia, 63–66, 64t
Acute tubular necrosis, 73–76, 74t
ADH, release of, from hypothalamus, 219, 220t
Adrenal cortex, 47–48
Albumin, intravenous, 98
Albuminuria, 22, 37, 42
Alcoholic ketosis, 268
Aldosterone, influence of, on sodium balance, 189
Alkalosis
  hypokalemic, 248
  metabolic, 197, 248, 274–276, 274f, 275t, 276t
  respiratory, 263, 264, 264t
  saline-resistant, 275
  saline-responsive, 275
Allopurinol therapy, 309
Alpha methyldopa, effect of, on serum creatinine, 59
Alport's syndrome, 42–43, 115–116

Aminoglycosides, factors affecting nephro-
toxicity of, 74, 74t
Amoxicillin, to treat urinary tract infection,
288, 289
Amyloidosis/neoplasia, 106–107, 107t
Analgesic nephropathy, 141
Anemia, 42
hypodromic microcytic, 143
Angiotensin, 228
Angiotensin converting enzyme (ACE)
inhibitors, 69, 72
Anion gap, as guide for classifying meta-
bolic acidosis, 264–265, 265f
Antibiotics, as cause of interstitial nephritis,
72
Antiglomerular basement membrane
(AGBM) disease, 92, 92t, 93
Anti-hypertensive therapy, for hypertensive
renal vascular disease, 162–163
Arteriography, 3t, 9, 11, 32
to diagnose renal artery stenosis, 47
Arthralgias, 138
Ascites, 1
Ascorbic acid
as cause of false-positive dipsticks, 32
effect of, on serum creatinine, 59
Aspirin, renal syndromes associated with,
141–142, 143t
Asymptomatic bacteriuria, 292
Atheroembolic renal artery disease,
166–167, 166t
Atherosclerosis, effect of, on renal function,
163
Atherosclerotic renal vascular diseases,
162t, 163–167, 165t
Autosomal dominant polycystic kidney
disease (ADPKD), 148, 150t
Azathioprine, for treatment of lupus
nephritis, 102
Azotemia, 31, 36, 38–40, 40t
acute, 18t
diagnostic approach to, 66–67, 67f, 68t
nonrenal causes of, 58–62, 59t
acute on chronic, 43–44, 44f
chronic, 18t
diagnostic approach to, 41t
distinguishing acute from chronic, 38–39,
40t
diagnostic approach to, 40–44, 41t, 43f,
44f
postrenal, 59–61, 60f, 61f, 62t
causes of, 61, 62t

prerenal
causes of, 62, 63t
versus acute renal failure, 63–66, 64t
Azotemic patient, renal ultrasonography in,
9–10

B

Bacterial cystourethritis, 287
Bacteriuria, 287
asymptomatic, 292
Balkan nephritis, 148
Balloon angioplasty, 8, 17f
Bartter's syndrome, 197, 247, 249, 275, 277
Basement membrane disease, thin, 31
Basement membrane theory, 105
Bence Jones proteins, 35, 36, 170
Bence Jones proteinuria, 38
Berger's disease, 31, 49–50, 171
Berry aneurysms, 148
Bicarbonate, organic acidosis treatment for,
268–269
Bilateral stenosis, 248
Bumetanide, 98

C

Calcium oxalate stones, 303
Calcium phosphate lithiasis, 307–308
Calcium phosphate stones, 307–308
Calculi, 30
Captopril, 99
"Captopril test," 47
Carcinoma, transitional cell, 30
Cefoxitin, 17
effect of, on serum creatinine, 59
Cell-mediated disease, 92, 92t, 93
Chlamydia urethritis, 289
Chlorambucil, for treatment of lupus
nephritis, 102
Chlorthalidone, 98
Cholestyramine, 306
Cimetidine, 16
effect of, on serum creatinine, 58
Cirrhosis, excess sodium in patients with,
202–203
Citrate, as cause of stone formation,
301–302
Computed tomography (CT), 2t, 5–6, 9,
11, 13f, 14f, 32, 60, 61f
Conn's syndrome, 45t, 46t, 48, 206

Continuous arteriovenous hemofiltration (CAVH), 82
Creatinine
  drugs which raise level of, 58–59
  nonrenal factors altering, 58, 59t
  production of, 14
  relationship between, and C$_{Cr}$, 20–21, 21f
Creatinine clearance (C$_{Cr}$), 14
  disadvantage of, 17
  interpretation of, 15–16
  relationship between creatinine and, 21f
Crohn's disease, 145
Cryoglobulinemia, 115, 168–169t, 170–171
CT. See Computed tomography
Cushing's syndrome, 45t, 46t, 47–48
Cyclophosphamide
  to treat lupus nephritis, 102, 103
  to treat Wegener's granulomatosis, 169
Cystinuria, 309
Cystography, 2t, 4, 9f
Cystolithiasis, assessment of, 3
Cystourethritis, 288–289
  bacterial, 287
Cystourethrogram, 5
Cystourethroscopy, 28
Cytotoxic therapy, in treating polyarteritis nodosa, 168–169

D

Denver shunt, 203
Diabetes insipidus
  etiologies of, 225, 225t
  nephrogenic, 24, 146
Diabetic ketoacidosis, 266, 268
Diabetic nephropathy, 103–106, 104f
Diffuse proliferative glomerulonephritis, 100–101t, 102
Digitalis, 228
Diuretics, 228
  in edematous therapy, 204–205
  renal potassium loss from, 246–247
  in treating nephrotic syndrome, 98
Diverticulosis, 148
Doxycycline, to treat urinary tract infections, 289
Drug-induced interstitial nephritis, 138–139, 138t, 141–142
DTPA, technetium-99m-tagged, 7
  nucleotide scan, 10
Dysuria, 28

E

ECV (total body sodium), depletion disorders, 195–197
  causes of, 196t
  diagnostic and therapeutic approach to patients with, 197–200, 199t
  signs and symptoms of, 195t
Edema, diagnostic approach to patients with, 206–207, 207t, 208, 208f
Edematous disorders, 200–201, 200t
  treatment of, 201–206
Empiric therapeutic trials, in classifying glomerulonephritis, 94
Enalapril, 99
Encephalopathy, 143
Enzymuria, 142
Eosinophilia, 166
Eosinophiluria, 138, 166
Erythromycin, to treat urinary tract infections, 289
Ethacrynic acid, 98
Excretory urogram (XU), 3
Extracorporeal shock wave lithotripsy (ESWL), principles of, 310

F

Fanconi's syndrome, 24, 146
FIASCO, 44
Focal proliferative glomerulonephritis, 100–101t, 101–102
Focal segmental glomerulosclerosis (FSG), 109–110
Furosemide, 98
  in treating hypernatremia, 231

G

Gastric stress ulceration, prophylaxis for, 81–82
Gastrointestinal fluids, sodium and potassium concentration in, 245, 245t
Genitourinary tract, imaging techniques for, 1, 2–3t
Glomerular dysfunction, measurement of, 21–22
Glomerular filtration rate (GFR), 187–189
  formula for estimating, 21
  measurement of, 12–14
Glomerular hemodynamics, 68–69, 72
Glomerular proteinuria, 36

Glomerulonephritis, 30, 42, 100–101t,
102–103
acute, 72
acute proliferative, 116–117
case discussions, 125–128
case presentations, 89–91
chronic, 120–121
clinical classification of, 94, 98t
diagnostic approach to, 121–125, 122f,
123f, 124f, 125f
diffuse proliferative, 100–101t, 102
focal proliferative, 100–101t, 101–102
focal segmental, 109–110
histologic classification of, 93–94, 96–97t
immune classification of, 92–93, 92t
infectious, 114
membranoproliferative, 43, 112–113, 118
membranous, 100–101t, 102, 107,
110–112, 111t
drugs associated with, 107, 108t
mesangioproliferative (IgA), 100–101t,
110, 117–118, 171
nephritic syndrome, 113
Alport's syndrome, 115–116
hereditary nephritis, 115–116
idiopathic, 116–118
infectious glomerulonephritis, 114
systemic lupus erythematosus, 114
vasculitis, 115
nephrotic syndrome, 94–95, 98–99
amyloidosis/neoplasia, 106–107, 107t
diabetic nephropathy, 103–106, 104f
idiopathic, 108–113
systemic lupus erythematosus, 100–103
rapidly progressive, 118–120
causes of, 119, 119t
Glomerulopathy, 42
Glomerulus
clinical evaluation of, 12–17, 20–22, 20f
functions of, 12, 20t
Glucocorticoid deficiency, 224
Glycosuria, 24
Goodpasture's syndrome, 72, 93, 119–120
Granulomatosis, Wegener's, 115, 168–169t,
169–170

H

Heart failure, factors contributing to hyponatremia in patients with chronic,
227–228, 228t

Hematuria, 18t, 22, 24, 28, 36, 287
diagnostic approach to, 32, 33f
etiology, 28, 29t, 30–32
Hemodynamics, glomerular, 68–69, 72
Hemoglobinuria, as cause of false-positive
dipsticks, 32
Hemolytic uremic syndromes, 115, 172
Henderson equation, 262
Henoch-Schönlein purpura, 115, 171
Hereditary nephritis, 42–43, 115–116
Hippuran, 6–7
Hippuran scanning, 6–7, 60–61
Hydrogen ion concentration
Henderson equation for, 262
relation of, to pH, 263t
Hyercalcemia, with hypercalciuria, 306t
Hyperaldosteronism, 45t, 46t, 48, 206
primary, 201
Hyperalimentation, influence of, on
prognosis of acute renal
failure, 82–83
Hypercalcemia, hypercalciuria without,
306t
Hypercalciuria, 146
and formation of calcium oxalate stones,
303, 306t
with hypercalcemia, 306t
without hypercalcemia, 306t
Hypercapnea, 275
Hyperchloremic acidosis, 24, 42, 265, 268
Hypercholesterolemia, 95
Hypercoagulable, 95
Hyperfiltration theory, 105
Hypergammaglobulinemia, and lowering of
serum sodium, 220
Hyperglycemia, and lowering of serum
sodium, 220
Hyperkalemia, 24, 42, 106
causes of, 249, 250t, 251
diagnostic approach to patients with, 251,
252f, 253
resulting from shift of potassium, 241,
241t
treatment of, 253–255, 254f
Hyperlipidemia, 95
and lowering of serum sodium, 220
Hypernatremia, 24, 221, 225–226, 225t
causes of, 225
with high total body sodium, 231
with low total body sodium, 229
as reflection of hyperosmolarity, 217
treatment of, 225–226

Hyperosmolarity, 217, 218
Hyperoxaluria, 145
  and formation of calcium oxalate stones, 303, 306
Hyperparathyroidism, 146
Hypersensitivity vasculitis, 115, 168–169t, 170
Hypertension, 18t, 31, 36, 42, 145
  adrenal cortex, 47–48
  case studies, 49–52
  causes of, 44, 45t
  effect of, on renal functions, 162–63
  pheochromocytoma, 45t, 46t, 48–49
  renal artery stenosis, 45, 45t, 46t, 47
  renal parenchymal disease, 45t, 46t, 47
  renovascular, 248
Hypertensive IVP, 3
Hypertriglyceridemia, 95
Hyperuricemia, 42
Hyperuricosuria, 308
  and formation of calcium oxalate stones, 306
Hypoalbuminemia, 206, 208
  therapy for, 203–204
Hypoaldosteronism, hyporeninemic, 106, 251
Hypochromic microcytic anemia, 143
Hypocitraturia, and formation of calcium oxalate stones, 306–307
Hypocomplementemia, 166, 171
Hypokalemia, 268
  causes of, 241, 241t, 244–247, 244t, 245t, 246f
  diagnostic approach to patients with, 246f, 247–249
  with metabolic alkalosis, 248
Hypokalemic alkalosis, 248
Hyponatremia, 22t, 220, 221, 223–225, 224t
  diagnostic and therapeutic approach to, 231
  drugs that cause, 223t
  with high total body sodium, 227–229, 228t
  with low total body sodium, 226–227
  as reflection of hypo-osmolarity, 217
Hypo-osmolarity, 217
Hyporeninemic hypoaldosteronism, 166, 251
Hyposthenuria, 23–24
Hypothalamus, ADH release from, 219, 220t
Hypothyroidism, 224
Hypovolemia, and stimulation of thirst, 218

I

Imaging techniques
  for genitourinary tract, 1, 2–3t
  problem-oriented approach to renal, 8–9, 18–19t
Immune complex disease, 92–93, 92t
Immune disorders, presentation as interstitial nephritis, 140
Immunoglobulin A (IgA) nephropathy, 31, 49–50, 171
Indium, 3t
Indium-tagged white blood cell (WBC) study, 7
Interstitium, 22–24
Intraurinary tract gas, detection of, 3
Intravenous digital subtraction angiography, to diagnose renal artery stenosis, 47
Intravenous pyelogram (IVP), 3, 9, 10
  to diagnose renal artery stenosis, 47
  hypertensive, 3
  with voiding and postvoid films, 2t
Inulin, clearance formula for, 13
Inulin infusion, 13

J

Jaffé reaction, effect of, on serum creatinine, 59
Juvenile nephronophthisis, 149

K

Kaliuresis, 247
Kayexalate, in treating hyperkalemia, 254
Ketoacidosis
  diabetic, 266, 268
  starvation, 266, 268
Ketosis, alcoholic, 266, 268
Kimmelstiel-Wilson disease, 93
KUB (abdominal film), 1, 2t, 3

L

Lactic acidosis, 266
Lead exposure, chronic, 142–143
Lead nephropathy, 142–143
Leukemia, myelogenous, 35
Leukocyte esterase, detection of, in urine, 287
LeVeen's shunt, 203
Light-chain nephropathy, 146–147

"Loop diuretics," and hyponatremia with high total body sodium, 227, 228t
Lupus nephritis, 102
  histologic varieties and clinical features of, 100–101t
  treatment of, 102–103
Lysozymuria, 35
Lytic lesions, assessment of, 3

M

Macroglobulinemia, Waldenström's, 147
Medical nephrectomy, 99
Medullary cystic disease (MCD), 148–149, 150t
Medullary sponge kidney (MSK), 149, 150t
Membranoproliferative glomerulonephritis, 43, 112–113, 118
Membranous glomerulonephritis, 100–101t, 102, 107, 110–112, 111t
  drugs associated with, 107, 108t
Mesangioproliferative glomerulonephritis, 100–101, 110, 117–118, 171
Metabolic acid base disorders
  case discussions, 279–281
  case presentations of, 259–262
  common etiologies of, 267
  diagnostic approach to, 276–278, 277f
  treatment for, 268
Metabolic acidosis, 42, 197, 264–266, 265f, 268
  diagnostic approach to, 269, 270f
Metabolic alkalosis, 197, 274–276, 274f, 276t
  generation or maintenance of, 275t
  hypokalemia with, 248
Metabolic theory, 105
Microangiopathic renal vascular disease
  hemolytic uremic syndrome, 171–173, 172t
  scleroderma, 173
  sickle cell nephropathy, 174
Microcirculation, diseases of, 73
Microhematuria, 105–106, 142
Mineralocorticoid activity, renal potassium loss as consequence of excess, 245
Mineralocorticoid escape, 189, 190f, 201, 248
Minimal change disease, 108–109
Mixed acid base disturbances, 264, 278–279, 278t
Monoclonal immunoglobulins, 170

Multiple myeloma. *See also* Myeloma kidney
  presentation of, as interstitial nephritis, 140
  renal syndromes associated with, 146, 147f
Myelogenous leukemia, 35
Myeloma kidney, 146–147, 146f, 147t. *See also* Multiple myeloma
Myoglobinuria, 32, 35

N

N-acetylated procainamide (NAPA), 82
Nail-patella, 147
Necrosis, renal
  acute tubular, 73–76, 74t
  papillary, 142
Nephrectomy, medical, 99
Nephritic syndrome, 30, 113
  Alport's syndrome, 115–116
  causes of, 113, 113t, 114t
  hereditary nephritis, 115–116
  idiopathic, 116–118
  infectious glomerulonephritis, 114
  systemic lupus erythematosus, 114
  vasculitis, 115
Nephritis
  Balkan, 148
  hereditary, 42–43, 115–116
  interstitial, 72–73
    acute, 136–140, 137t, 138t
    case discussions of, 154–156
    case presentations of, 131–137
    chronic, 51, 136, 140–149, 137t
    diagnostic approach to, 137t, 149, 151–152, 151f, 152f, 153t, 154
    drug-induced, 138–139, 138t, 141–142
    hereditary diseases associated with, 147–149
    lupus, 100–101t, 102–103
    tubulointerstitial, 35
Nephrocalcinosis, 3, 145–146
Nephrogenic diabetes insipidus, 24, 146
Nephrolithiasis, 145
  assessment of, 3
  calcium oxalate stones, 303
    hypercalciuria, 303, 306t
    hyperoxaluria, 303, 306
    hyperuricosuria, 306
    hypocitraturia, 306–307
  calcium phosphate stones, 307–308

Nephrolithiasis (Continued)
case discussion of, 313, 315–316
case presentations of, 297–301
causes of, 302–303, 302t, 304–305t
cystinuria, 309
diagnostic approach to, 312t, 313, 314f
evaluation of patient with, 309
general advice for patients with, 311t
medical approach to, 311–312, 311t
serial evaluation of, 3
stone formation, 301–302
struvite stones, 308
uric acid stones, 308–309
urologic approach to, 310–311
Nephrologic syndromes, associated with
nonsteroidal anti-inflammatory drugs
(NSAIDs), 74–75
Nephronophthisis, juvenile, 149
Nephropathy
analgesic, 141
chronic oxalate, 145
chronic urate, 145
diabetic, 103–106, 104f
immunoglobulin A, 31, 49–50, 171
interstitial, 24
light-chain, 146–147
sickle cell, 174
uric acid, 140
Nephrostolithotomy, percutaneous, 310
Nephrotic proteinuria, 37, 99, 206, 208
Nephrotic-range proteinuria, 37
Nephrotic syndrome, 30, 36, 94–95, 98–99
amyloidosis/neoplasia, 106–107, 107t
causes of, 99, 99t
diabetic nephropathy, 103–106, 104f
idiopathic, 108–113
systemic lupus erythematosus, 100–102t
treatment of, 98–99
Nephrotomography, 1, 3, 6f
Neuropathy, peripheral, 143
Nitrite, detection of, in urine, 287
Nitrogen mustard, for treatment of lupus
nephritis, 102
Nonabsorbable anions, as cause of hypokalemia, 245–246
Nonoliguria, versus oliguria, 81
Nonsteriodal anti-inflammatory drugs
(NSAIDS)
as cause of acute renal failure, 72
and hyperkalemic syndrome, 251
nephrologic syndromes associated with,
74–75

in treating nephrotic syndrome, 99
Normal total body sodium, isolated disorders of water balance in patients
with, 220–221, 221f, 223
Nuclear scanning, in diagnosing postrenal
azotemia, 60–61

O

Obstruction, 19t
Oliguria, versus nonoliguria, 81
Organic acidosis, 265, 266–267
Orthophosphates, 307
Orthostatic proteinuria, 37, 38
Osmolar gap, 217
causes of, 217, 217t
Osmolarity, 216–217
Osteodystrophy, assessment of, 3
Osteolysis, idiopathic multicentric, 148
Overflow proteinuria, 35–36
Oxalate, dietary sources of, 307
Oxypurinol stones, 309

P

Percutaneous nephrostolithotomy, 310
Peripheral neuropathy, 143
Peritoneal gas, detection of, 3
pH, relation of hydrogen ion concentration
(H+) to, 263t
Pheochromocytoma, 45t, 46t, 48–49
Plasmapheresis, 103
Polyarteritis nodosa (PAN), 115, 167–169,
168–169t
Polyclonal immunoglobulins, 170
Polycystic kidney disease, 14f
Polydipsia, psychogenic, 223
Postrenal azotemia, 59–61, 60f, 61f, 62t
causes of, 61, 62t
Potassium, renal handling of, 240f,
242–243, 242f, 243t
Potassium balance disorders
case discussion of, 255–257
case presentations of, 237–239
hypokalemia, 267
causes of, 241, 241t, 244–247, 244t,
245t, 246f
diagnostic approach to patients with,
246f, 247—249
with metabolic alkalosis, 248

Potassium excretion, 240f, 242
Potassium homeostasis, 239, 240f, 241, 241t, 242
Potassium secretion, 242–243, 242t
  nonspecific factors affecting, 243, 243t
Potassium shift, causes of, 241, 241t, 249
Prerenal azotemia
  causes of, 62, 63t
  versus acute renal failure, 63–66, 64t
Progressive systemic sclerosis (PSS), 173
Prostatitis, 290
Protein, determining proper amount of dietary, in treating nephrotic syndrome, 98
Proteinuria, 18t, 22, 24, 31, 34–35, 34f, 35t
  diagnostic approach to, 38, 39f
  glomerular, 36
  nephrotic, 37, 99, 206, 208
  orthostatic, 37, 38
  overflow, 35–36
  tubulointerstitial, 35, 36–37
Pseudohyperkalemia, 249, 251
Psoas obliteration, 1
Psychogenic polydipsia, 223
Pulmonary artery wedge pressure (PAWP), 67
Pulse methylprednisolone therapy, 120
Purpura, Henoch-Schönlein, 115, 171
Pyelography, renal, 2t, 4, 8f, 9, 10, 28, 30
Pyelonephritis, 287
  acute, 139, 288
    as cause of acute renal failure, 73
  chronic, 144, 145
  subclinical, 288
Pyuria, 24, 287

R

Radiographs, to diagnose renal artery stenosis, 45, 47
Radionuclide scanning, 2t, 6–7
Raynaud's phenomenon, 171
RBC cast, 30, 30f, 31f
Renal acid excretion, components of, 271f
Renal arteriography, 8, 15f, 16f, 17f
Renal artery embolism, 165–166, 165t
Renal artery stenosis, 15f, 16f, 45, 45t, 46t, 47
Renal biopsy, 32
  use of, in classifying glomerulonephritis, 93–94

Renal cysts and tumors, detection of, 3
Renal failure. *See also* Acute renal failure
  chronic, and excess sodium, 200–201
  urinary tract infections with, 292–293
Renal imaging techniques, problem-oriented approach to, 8–9, 18–19t
Renal insufficiency, 3
Renal mass, 19t
Renal papillary necrosis, 142
Renal parenchyma, assessment of, 3
Renal parenchymal disease (RPD), 45t, 46t, 47
Renal tubular acidosis (RTA), 269
  clinical features of, 271t
  common causes of, 272t
  distal, 146, 247, 273
  mixed type, 273
  proximal, 247, 269–273
Renal tubular cell casts, 24
Renal tubules, 20t
  clinical evaluation of, 22–24
  functions of, 22
Renal ultrasonogram, 5, 10f, 11, 11f, 12f
Renal vascular disease
  hypentensive, 161–163, 162t
  microangiopathic, 171–174, 172t
Renal vein thrombosis (RVT), 95, 174–175
  signs of, 95
  tendency for recurrence, 95
Renal venography, 95, 174–175
Renovascular hypertension, 3, 248
Respiratory acidosis
  causes of, 264, 264t
  effects of, 263
Respiratory alkalosis
  causes of, 264, 264t
  effects of, 263
Retinopathy, 106
Retrograde pyelography, 2t, 4, 8f, 9, 10
Retroperitoneal gas, detection of, 3
Rhabdomyolysis, 21, 35

S

Saline-resistant alkalosis, 275
Saline-responsive alkalosis, 275
Sarcoidosis, 146
Sclerosis, progressive systemic, 173
Sclerotic lesions, assessment of, 3
Scleroderma, 173
Serum osmolarity, formula for, 217

SIADH. *See* Syndrome of inappropriate
    ADH secretion (SIADH)
Sickle cell nephropathy, 174
Sodium balance, control of, 187–190, 188f,
    189t, 190f, 191f, 192, 193f, 194–195,
    194f
Sodium balance disorders
    case discussions, 208–211
    case presentations of, 183–187
    diagnostic approach to patients with
        edema, 206–207
    edematous disorders, 200–201
        treatment of, 201–206
    sodium (ECV) depletion disorders
        diagnostic and therapeutic approach to
            patients with, 197–200, 199t
        signs and symptoms of, 195t
Starling forces, 192
Starvation ketoacidosis, 268
Stenosis, bilateral, 248
Steroids, for treatment of lupus nephritis,
    102
Stone formation, 301–302
Struvite stones, 308
Subclinical pyelonephritis, 288
Syndrome of inappropriate ADH secretion
    (SIADH)
    causes of, 224, 224t
    diagnosis of, 224, 224t
Systemic lupus erythematosus, 100–103, 114

T

Technetium-99m-tagged DPTA, 7
    nucleotide scan, 10
Thiazides, 98
Thirst, 218
Thrombotic thrombocytopenic purpura
    (TTP), 172–173
Total body sodium. *See* ECV (total body
    sodium) depletion disorders
Triamterene, 309
Trimethoprim, 16
    effect of, on serum creatinine, 58
Trimethoprim-sulfamethoxazole (TMP/
    SMZ), to treat urinary tract
    infection, 288, 289, 290, 291
Tubular cell injury, 140
Tubular dysfunction, failure to reabsorb
    filtered water as sign of, 23
Tubular reabsorption, indication of, 23

Tubular toxicity/obstruction, 145–146
    in interstitial nephritis, 140
Tubulointerstitial nephritis, 35
Tubulointerstitial proteinuria, 35, 36–37

U

Ultrasonography, 2t
    in diagnosing postrenal azotemia, 60, 60f
    renal, 5, 10f, 11, 11f, 12f
Urea, nonrenal factors altering, 58, 59t
Uremic acidosis, 266, 268
Ureteral catheterization, 31–32
Urethral diverticulum, 28
Urethritis, 287
Uric acid nephropathy, 140
Uric acid stones, 308–309
Urinalysis (UA), in diagnosing urinary tract
    infection, 287
Urinary abnormalities
    asymptomatic, 52
    azotemia, 38–40, 40t
        diagnostic approach, 40–44, 41t, 43f,
            44f
    case discussions, 49–52
    case presentations, 25–28
    hematuria, 28
        diagnostic approach to, 32, 33f
        etiology, 28, 29t, 30–32
    hypertension, 44
        adrenal cortex, 47–48
        pheochromocytoma, 45t, 46t, 48–49
        renal artery stenosis, 45t, 46t, 47
        renal parenchymal disease (RPD), 45t,
            46t, 47
    proteinuria, 34–35, 34f, 35t
        diagnostic approach to, 38, 39f
Urinary protein electrophoresis, 37
Urinary sodium (UA)
    as indicator of tubular reabsorptive
        capacity, 23
    sensitivity of, 23
Urinary supersaturation, as cause of stone
    formation, 301
Urinary tract infections (UTIs), 19t
    catheter-related, 291
    complicated, 290–291
    diagnosis of, 285, 286t, 287
    recurrent, 291
    uncomplicated, 293–294, 293f
    with renal failure, 292–293

Urinary tract infection syndromes
  acute pyelonephritis, 288
  case discussion of, 294–296
  case presentations of, 283–285
  chlamydia urethritis, 289
  cystourethritis, 288–289
  prostatitis, 290
  subclinical pyelonephritis, 288
  urinary tract infections
    asymptomatic bacteriuria, 292
    catheter-related, 291
    complicated, 290–291
    recurrent, 291
    urinary tract infection with renal
      failure, 292–293
  vaginitis, 290
Urine collection, need for timed, in creatine
    clearance test, 17
Urine culture, in diagnosing urinary tract
    infection, 287
Urine immunoelectrophoresis, 37
Urine sediment, examination of, in diag-
    nosis of urinary tract infection, 287
Urogram, excretory, 3

V

Vaginitis, 287, 290
Vascular disease of kidney, 73
  atherosclerotic renal vascular diseases,
      162t, 163–167, 165t
  case discussions of, 177–180
  case presentations of, 157–161
  diagnostic approach to, 175, 176f,
      177–178
  hypertensive renal vascular disease,
      161–163, 162t
  microangiopathic renal vascular disease
    hemolytic uremic syndrome, 171–173,
        172t
    scleroderma, 173
    sickle cell nephropathy, 174
  renal vein thrombosis, 174–175
  systemic vasculitic syndromes, 167,
      168–169t
    cryoglobulinemia, 168–169t, 170–171
    hypersensitivity vasculitis, 168–169t, 170

polyarteritis nodosa (PAN), 167–169,
    168–169t
Wegener's granulomatosis, 168–169t,
    169–170
Vasculitis, 115
  systemic, 72, 119, 167, 168–169t
    cryoglobulinemia, 168–169t, 170–171
    hypersensitivity vasculitis, 168–169t,
        170
    polyarteritis nodosa (PAN), 167–169,
        168–169t
    Wegener's granulomatosis, 168–169t,
        169–170
Venography, renal, 95, 174–175
Venous digital subtraction angiography
    (DSA), 10
Vesicoureteral reflux (VUR), 144–145
von Hippel Lindau disease, 147

W

Waldenström's macroglobulinemia, 147
Water, renal handling of, 218–219, 218f
Water balance, control of, 217–220, 218f
Water balance disorders, 216–217
  case discussion of, 231–235
  case presentations of, 213–217
  hypernatremia, 225–226, 225t
    causes of, 225
    with high total body sodium, 231
    with low total body sodium, 229
    treatment of, 225–226
  hyponatremia, 222t, 223–225, 224t
    with high total body sodium, 227–229,
        228t
    with low total body sodium, 226–227
  in patients with normal total body
      sodium, 220–221, 221f, 223
  simultaneous disorders of water and total
      body sodium, 226
Wegener's granulomatosis, 115, 168–169t,
    169–170
White blood count (WBC), 24

X

Xanthine stones, 309
XU *See* Excretory urogram